DELAVIER'S
SCULPTING ANATOMY
FOR WOMEN

DELAVIER'S SCULPTING ANATOMY FOR WOMEN

Core, Butt, and Legs

Frédéric Delavier • Jean-Pierre Clémenceau

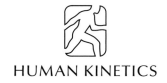

HUMAN KINETICS

CONTENTS

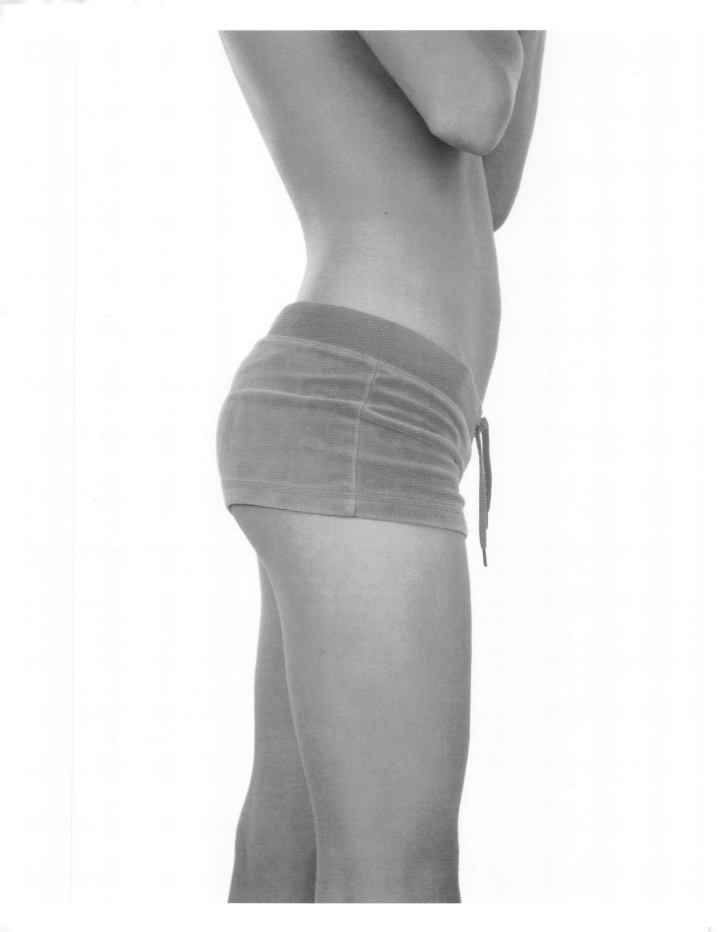

Women who are concerned about their figures dream of having a flat belly and a sculpted butt, yet these crucial areas often lack tone and firmness.

Frédéric Delavier, renowned author of books about the anatomy of movement, and Jean-Pierre Clémenceau, well-known coach to international celebrities, have combined their expertise in creating a new workout program specifically designed for women who want to sculpt the core, butt, and legs in just three months.

The authors present exercises that are targeted for each part of the body to be developed. Each exercise is richly illustrated with photographs and anatomical drawings that will help you quickly and precisely visualize the muscle groups that you wish to work. Delavier and Clémenceau specialize in proper positioning and correct breathing techniques. For each exercise, they detail the number of sets and repetitions you should do and give you critical advice and warnings so that you can perform the exercises correctly and safely. They also show you how to breathe correctly during the exercise so you can increase the effectiveness and achieve improved muscle tone.

To obtain fast results, you should do at least a minimum amount of cardiorespiratory work so that you do not become winded during workouts. The heart is the body's motor, and it will not be able to sustain long-term physical effort if it is in poor condition. The work to get your heart into shape can be the same for every person, regardless of age, but various options are presented to suit your ability. This is why, for the same exercise, you may do sets of 10, 15, or even 20 repetitions.

To ensure each exercise you do is as effective as possible, you need to avoid relying on other muscle groups to compensate for weaknesses in targeted muscle groups. Improving your body's mobility and ease of movement will help you achieve this.

Exercise alone will not help you lose weight; balanced nutrition that is adapted to your life-style will do the trick. No more diets! In this book, you will learn to adjust your food intake as a function of your physical activity and your body's energy needs. The wealth of advice from a bodybuilding specialist and a professional coach will give you all the tools you need to sculpt a flat belly, a sexy, firm butt, and toned legs in just a few weeks.

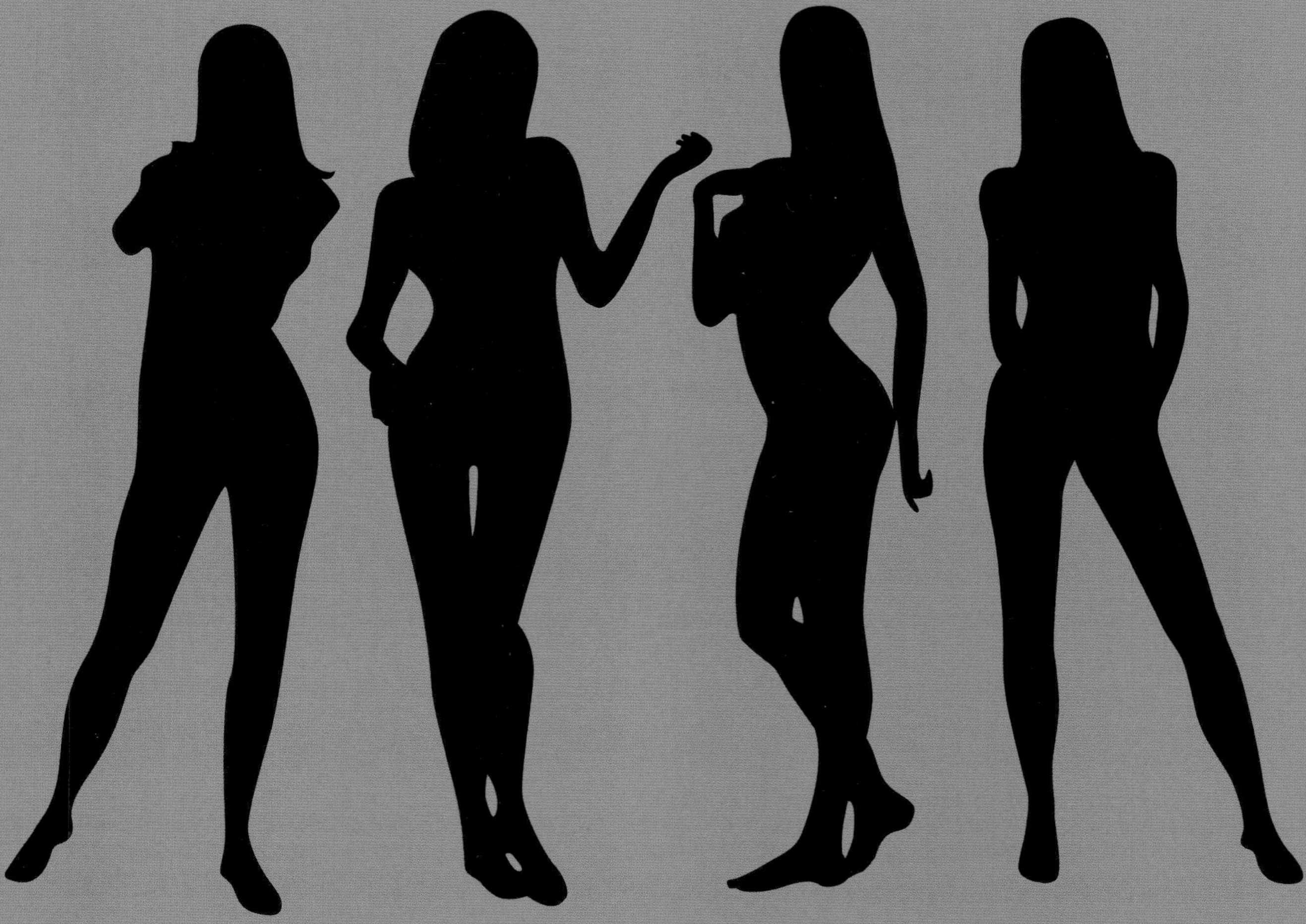

YOUR MISSION
A Flat Belly
and a Sexy Butt

in 3 months

FIVE TIPS
TO GET YOU STARTED

Before starting your workout program, carefully read the following five tips. They will help you get started correctly and give you all the tools you need for success.

(1) MOTIVATION IS ESSENTIAL

Are you uncomfortable with your body? Do you feel restricted or even unable to do the things you want? Would you like to change your body and improve your self-confidence? There is always a deciding moment that pushes a woman to take that step and begin doing a physical activity or resume a lapsed exercise regimen. Striving to improve well-being and appearance and alleviate strain, stress, and even depression are among the most common reasons for exercising.

There are multiple steps, but whether you want to improve your quality of life or improve your figure, your motivation will be the driving force behind your physical activity. The pleasure you get from working out combined with the effort you put in and the visible results will be your fuel. You will feel better and more toned, have better cardiorespiratory endurance, and lose weight and keep it off. These results will keep you motivated to achieve your goal of getting back in shape. Each day, not only will you notice the positive results of your tenacity, but everyone around you will notice your newfound well-being.

When you decide to do any kind of physical activity, you make the choice to accept a new way of life. You decide to change your habits by making the time to go to the gym or work out at home using the exercises in this book. This also means rethinking your diet, since it is impossible to achieve physical well-being, beat stress, and reduce tension on your muscles and joints while eating an imbalanced diet. But rest assured, if you continue working hard, you will see results and your motivation to keep exercising will increase.

How many times should you work out each week?

Certainly the time you have available to exercise each week depends on your obligations and your schedule. Know that if you can work out only once each week, that is still better than not working out at all. Two workouts are a good minimum, and the ideal is three workouts each week. However, if you have a ton of energy and enthusiasm to start, just be careful not to overdo it. Too much motivation, which is very common when beginning to exercise again, can quickly falter due to fatigue from overtraining. Pace yourself so that you can persevere and obtain your desired results. One final piece of advice: At a minimum, try to schedule your workouts every other day so that your body has a chance to recover between workouts.

② IT'S NEVER TOO LATE TO RESHAPE YOUR BODY

Women who are over 30 who have avoided the slightest physical activity throughout life and want to start exercising always ask me (Jean-Pierre) the same question: "Is it too late for me to develop my muscles?" The answer is no, because even if you have not used your muscles very much, they are still there, just waiting to give their best effort. So do not hesitate to start on the path to getting into shape, even if you have not exercised in years.

Muscle weakness makes the entire figure seem softer. Skin, which can expand, takes on the shape of the muscle, and of course, the weaker the muscle is, the more the skin tends to collapse. Over time, skin loses its elasticity; thus there's a need to maintain a certain amount of muscle tone or to redevelop muscle. Still, the later you begin, the longer and more difficult strength training will be. It will take two to three years for a 60-year-old person to develop the triceps muscle, while a 30-year-old can do it in two to three months. And for all those 50-year-olds who are despairing because they never exercised when they were younger, know that you can build muscle even up to age 70. So, to your weights! But be careful to adjust your workout routine to match your age and abilities.

Some of my students are 70, 75, even 80 years old. Maybe they exercised all their lives, or perhaps they only started around age 40, but they continue to train regularly. Of course, I would never ask them to do 30 push-ups to develop the muscles in their

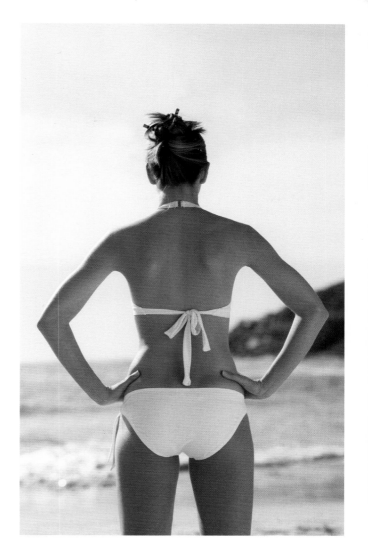

back! Even if they are in great shape, their hearts cannot tolerate the intensity of certain exercises. I will share with you an anecdote about one of my students, 70 years old, whom I train regularly. She played tennis her whole life but had to stop a few years ago because of severe back pain. Three years ago, we began working to develop her buttocks, back, and core muscles. Today, not only has she begun playing tennis again, but she is beating some of her friends who used to be stronger than she was! You can imagine how happy she is.

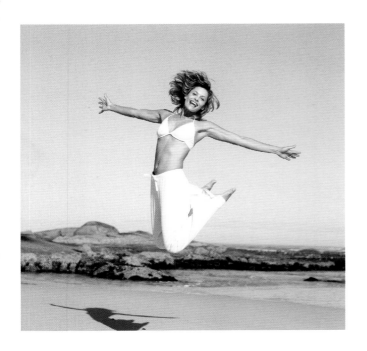

"I have given myself a second chance at youth," she confided to me. Yet she hates working out. Those few exercises and the well-being she gained from them changed her mind. Her muscles are stronger, and her bones are too because, like muscles, bones grow stronger with physical activity.

Advantages of Working Out at Home

There are many advantages to exercising at home. First, it is more practical (you save time and you can work out whenever you want to), and it is more economical since you do not have to pay the high cost of a gym membership. Using this book and the professional advice from leading coaches, you will learn that exercising at home is just as effective as going to a gym. Your concentration will only improve during a quicker and more productive workout.

One simple tip is to film your workout. Even if you exercise in front of a mirror, seeing yourself on video will help you truly determine whether or not you are performing the exercises correctly. This way you can correct yourself and keep improving.

③ EXERCISE FOR YOUR HEALTH

Your doctor has probably advised you to do some exercise to maintain heart health, improve blood circulation, and protect your overall health. Indeed, today it is difficult not to know that a minimum amount of physical activity is required for maintaining health, especially since the risk of cardiovascular disease and diabetes increases in people who are overweight. A person who does not exercise will lose nearly a quarter of her muscle mass between ages 35 and 70. But if the body is worked regularly, it becomes more resistant and does not tire as easily. Working your body regularly will increase your resistance and help you maintain good physical and mental health. Maintaining a healthy weight and staying active are the only secrets to longevity.

④ LISTEN TO YOUR BODY

We must emphasize that exercising to get into shape applies only to people who are able to exercise and have no special physical conditions. We are speaking especially to people who have back problems or who have muscle or joint problems.

The human body is so well made that it always gives a warning before a serious problem develops. Unfortunately, many people do not know—or do not want to know—how to interpret these signals. You might ignore the pain in your shoulder that indicates a tendon problem, which will sideline you for three weeks. Lower back pain is preceded by signals that you might deliberately choose to ignore. Try to listen to your body and identify any pain you feel.

Recurring pain indicates muscle spasms or nerve inflammation. If in doubt, stop exercising and see a doctor before resuming. Remember that it is very dangerous to work a part of the body that hurts or a muscle that is having spasms. When you feel that your body is stiff and tight, this means your muscles are shortened and blood is not flowing smoothly. Working the muscles will only accentuate the compression and the contraction of the fibers. Before any muscle work, you should do a few stretches to relax your limbs and lengthen your muscles. Once you have achieved good mobility in your body, you can begin working on getting into shape.

I try to pay close attention to what my body is telling me. One time I had pain in my abdomen, and, despite the fact that I know my body extremely well, I could not identify the cause. I had an ultrasound done immediately, and it was only a small tear in the fibers of the abdominal muscles as a result of too much exercise. It was a classic mistake of doing too much at the end of a workout. My body was already tired and it reacted badly. You see, even I am not immune to this kind of mistake!

⑤ EXERCISE FOR BEAUTY

Though regular physical activity is certainly the best way to maintain a small waist and slim legs, it is pointless to jump on the scale after your first few gym sessions or workouts because you will risk disappointment. You should know—and

I tell my clients this each day if I see that they are discouraged—that exercise will not make you lose weight. It is diet, and diet alone, that determines weight. At the end of a month of working out, when my students do not notice any changes in their appearance, I explain to them that no miracle can happen without two or three workouts every week for a minimum of two months.

Rest assured that by doing regular and powerful exercises, fat will be transformed into muscle. But it is better not to have your judgment clouded by the scale, because muscle weighs more than fat. This is why a person who starts exercising can seem thinner and more toned and still weigh exactly the same or even slightly more. Do not forget that the time it takes your body to adapt to an exercise routine is different for each person. Two people who are the same age can do the same exercises on the same schedule, yet they will not reshape their figures at the same speed or in the same way.

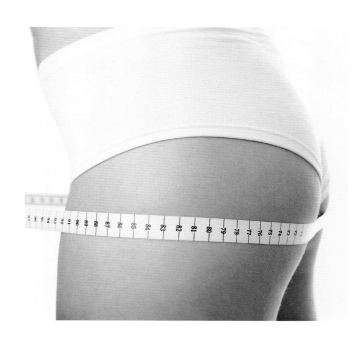

NUTRITION: THE FOUNDATION OF HEALTH

Before discussing questions about health and physical condition, with all the right exercises to reshape your body, we must highlight the importance of nutritional balance. In fact, you cannot have well-being and vitality without a simple daily nutrition plan. We will not give you a list of forbidden foods, because there is no such thing. Similarly, we will not advise you to follow any particular diet, since your body needs sugar and fat, but within reason and at certain times.

This diet could be summed up as a little bit of everything, but it's not as simple as that. To avoid draconian diets that perturb the body and interfere with metabolism, you must listen to your body and its needs and learn to nourish yourself depending on your age and your activity level.

RULES OF NUTRITION

RETHINK YOUR DIET AND YOUR MEALS

Remember that as you age, your body will not react the way it used to. A good diet, combined with exercise, will become the prerequisite for maintaining a fit and firm physique for as long as possible. After age 30, metabolism changes and alters your digestion, a peculiarity that especially affects women. Since cells secrete fewer digestive juices, food is absorbed more slowly and less easily. So you will need to reconsider the food you eat and the timing of your meals while limiting the consumption of certain foods that are very rich and hard to digest, especially in the evening. We will revisit this topic and give you some basic rules that are easy to memorize. They will help you fight the tendency to do exactly the opposite of what your body needs regarding nutrition, especially eating heavier and heavier meals throughout the day.

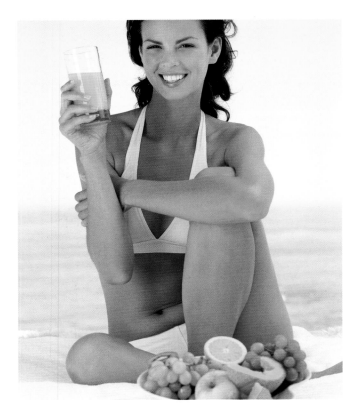

DAILY ENERGY AND CALORIE REQUIREMENTS

MALE	
SEDENTARY	2,400 calories/day
Protein	90 g
Fat	90 g
Carbohydrate	310 g
MODERATE ACTIVITY LEVEL	3,000 calories/day
Protein	100 g
Fat	90 g
Carbohydrate	450 g
HIGH ACTIVITY LEVEL	3,500 to 4,500 calories/day
Protein	110 to 120 g
Fat	95 to 115 g
Carbohydrate	470 to 800 g

FEMALE	
SEDENTARY	2,000 calories/day
Protein	75 g
Fat	75 g
Carbohydrate	250 g
MODERATE ACTIVITY LEVEL	2,300 to 2,500 calories/day
Protein	90 to 95 g
Fat	90 g
Carbohydrate	330 g
HIGH ACTIVITY LEVEL	3,000 to 3,500 calories/day
Protein	100 to 110 g
Fat	90 g
Carbohydrate	470 to 580 g

ENERGY USED DURING EXERCISE

When you put forth an intense physical effort, as during a long, serious workout, the cells in your body get most of the energy they need from fatty tissues—that is, from fat located under the skin.

If the intensity of the exercise increases, your muscles will require more fuel in order to react. So a process that burns carbohydrate and decreases the amount of fat burned will start. After a sustained effort lasting 30 to 40 minutes, your body will automatically start burning fat reserves.

BEWARE OF HUNGER AFTER A WORKOUT

You might have noticed that after a very hard workout you feel hungry. Indeed, after exercise, metabolism slows and weakens, the muscles relax, and the depletion of carbohydrate reserves triggers a sensation of hunger.

This is not the time to grab a sugary drink or a really fattening dessert. If you cannot wait for mealtime, eat one or two semiacidic fruits and some nonfat cottage cheese or a low-fat yogurt. You could even have an energy bar that will make you feel full without actually filling you up with too many calories. It is better to eat energy bars made with apples and grains rather than those made with dried fruit or chocolate.

SAMPLE MENU WITH LIGHT MEALS	
TOTAL FOR THE DAY: 1,605 CALORIES	
BREAKFAST: 510 calories	
Coffee or tea	0 cal.
(with sugar)	20 cal.
2 slices bread with low-fat butter	360 cal.
1 plain yogurt	65 cal.
1 glass orange juice	65 cal.
LUNCH: 400 calories	
1 fish filet (steamed or grilled, 3.5 oz, or 100 g)	90 cal.
Green vegetables (3.5 oz, or 100 g)	25 cal.
Green salad with low-fat dressing	45 cal.
Cheese (1 oz, or 30 g)	110 cal.
1 cup of custard	130 cal.
DINNER: 695 calories	
Plate of raw vegetables (4 oz, or 150 g)	165 cal.
Potato omelet (2 eggs and ~2 oz [50 g] potatoes)	195 cal.
Green salad with low-fat dressing	45 cal.
Piece of goat cheese	190 cal.
Low-fat cottage cheese	100 cal.

SAMPLE MENU WITH HEAVY MEALS	
TOTAL FOR THE DAY: 4,310 CALORIES	
BREAKFAST: 830 calories	
Coffee or tea	0 cal.
(with sugar)	20 cal.
1 croissant	205 cal.
2 slices buttered bread	400 cal.
1 glass orange juice	65 cal.
1 yogurt with fruit	140 cal.
LUNCH: 1,850 calories	
Avocado	360 cal.
1 slice of beef (5 oz, or 140 g)	310 cal.
1 serving of French fries (5 oz, or 140 g)	560 cal.
1 piece of goat cheese (1.5 oz, or 40 g)	190 cal.
2 scoops vanilla ice cream	230 cal.
2 glasses red wine	200 cal.
DINNER: 1,630 calories	
2 slices toast with hummus	400 cal.
Assortment of cold cuts	550 cal.
Potatoes au gratin (1 cup)	230 cal.
1 glass red wine	100 cal.
Green salad with dressing	75 cal.
1 fruit tart	275 cal.

Optimize Your Diet to Slim Your Waist

Low-carbohydrate diets are the most effective at accentuating inches lost around the waist. Sugar, as well as alcohol, promote the storage of fat around the waist. So it is a good idea to eat bread, pasta, rice, sweets, and pastries in moderation. Pay special attention to sweetened carbonated beverages (sodas), which are high in both sugar and caffeine. In fact, sodas promote the absorption of sugar, making them even more harmful to your health and waistline.

Nutritional Supplements for a Flat Belly

Nutritional supplements such as branched-chain amino acids (BCAAs) and calcium help to localize fat loss around the waist.

→ BCAAs include three essential amino acids (leucine, isoleucine, and valine). These three amino acids make up one-third of all muscle proteins. However, the human body does not have the necessary enzymes to manufacture them. You can meet your BCAA requirements only through diet or supplementation. BCAAs promote muscle strengthening, combat the storage of fat, stimulate the secretion of growth hormone (anti-fat),

support the secretion of a hunger-fighting hormone (leptin), and help overcome physical and mental fatigue during exercise and while dieting. You can find BCAAs in powdered form, in caplets or tablets, and as highly concentrated protein (whey, casein).

→ Calcium is a mineral most commonly found in dairy products, and it has an essential role in bone health. Recent scientific discoveries have shown that calcium has a basic action on fat. While dieting, you most likely do not meet your body's increasing need for calcium. One solution is to supplement, because including dairy products in a diet increases the amount of calories consumed. Calcium needs vary depending on your age (1.3 grams per day for adolescents, 1 gram for adults, 1.3 grams for people over 50). Ideally, you should consume two-thirds of your calcium at night and one-third in the morning. Be careful not to consume more than 2.5 grams per day.

NUTRIENTS THAT GIVE YOU ENERGY

• •

To be healthy, your body needs fuel. Protein, carbohydrate, and fat in your diet are essential nutrients that provide your body with the energy it needs.

PROTEIN (OR AMINO ACIDS)

Proteins vary according to the amino acids they contain. They are made up of carbon, oxygen, hydrogen, and nitrogen. Each molecule contains about 30 different amino acids. Life cannot exist without protein; it is essential for building the body because it repairs and maintain cells, and it helps in the proper assimilation of carbohydrate and fat.

Since cells cannot manufacture their own protein, these essential building blocks must come from your diet. Fibroblasts in the skin need protein to make the collagen fibers that provide elasticity

CLASSIFICATION OF FRUITS			
ACIDIC FRUITS (100 g = 3.5 oz)		**SEMIACIDIC FRUITS**	
Mandarin orange	10 cal.	Apricot	22 cal.
Lemon	20 cal.	Strawberries (100 g)	35 cal.
Grapefruit	40 cal.	Raspberries (100 g)	40 cal.
Orange	50 cal.	Peach	45 cal.
Blackcurrant (100 g)	41 cal.	Apple	52 cal.
Pineapple (100 g)	54 cal.	Pear	60 cal.
		Acidic grapes (white grapes, 100 g)	70 cal.
SWEET FRUITS		**STARCHY FRUITS**	
Mango (100 g)	64 cal.	Prune	26 cal.
Sweet apples and muscat grapes	70 cal.	Banana	90 cal.
Cherries (100 g)	77 cal.	Chestnuts (100 g)	180 cal.
Fresh fig	80 cal.	Dates and dried fruits	300 cal.
MELONS			
Melon (100 g)	27 cal.		
Watermelon (100 g)	30 cal.		

to the skin. Protein can be found in foods such as red meat, poultry, deli meats, milk, cheese, eggs, fish, and shellfish. Protein also plays a role in providing energy, and it contains a lot of calories. This means that while you are eating protein, you should consume less sugar and fat.

If you eat more protein than your body needs, then it will undergo a process of oxidation and be converted to fat. There are two kinds of protein: fibrous and globular. Fibrous protein is insoluble and makes up the structure of numerous tissues in your body such as hair, skin, muscles, tendons, and cartilage.

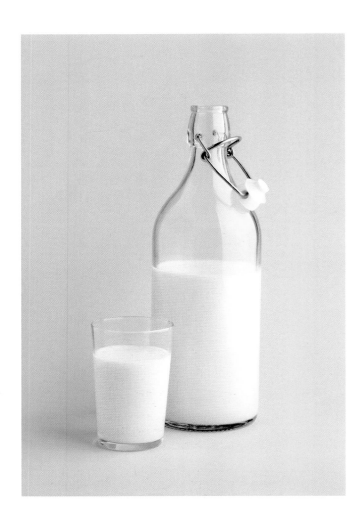

is burned, fat provides energy for your body (calories helpful in maintaining body temperature) and also serves as a solvent for certain elements of the body during fermentation. Excess saturated fat (animal fat and hydrogenated oil) leads to higher blood cholesterol levels and to excess weight. Foods that contain animal fat are butter, margarine, eggs, cooked or raw cheese, yogurt, deli meat, milk, fish, and red meat. Foods that contain vegetable fat are pasta, dried vegetables, nuts, almonds, flour, bread, and vegetable oils.

Fats can be divided into two groups: Saturated fat is solid, such as deli meat, dairy products, and eggs, while monounsaturated fat includes all fats that do not solidify at room temperature, such as vegetable, fish, avocado, and olive oil.

Finally, you should know that cholesterol is a type of fat, that there is no bad cholesterol in food, and that only your body along with faulty metabolism can produce it. So you should eat the following foods in moderation: egg yolks (make omelets with two whites and one yolk), giblets, butter, deli meats, and fatty cheeses.

Globular protein is soluble and starts biochemical reactions for numerous hormones such as growth hormone and antibodies.

FAT (OR FATTY ACIDS)

Fat is primarily made up of carbon, oxygen, and hydrogen. These are primarily fatty substances from animals or vegetables that contain numerous vitamins, especially vitamins A, B, and E. As it

CARBOHYDRATE

First and foremost, carbohydrate is a substance made of sugar and, like fat, is composed of carbon, oxygen, and hydrogen. Carbohydrate is an energy-providing nutrient that promotes endurance during intense physical exercise.

There are two categories of carbohydrate that are more or less quickly assimilated and burned by the body:

→ Fast-acting sugar (or simple carbohydrate) that is quickly absorbed: fruit, jams, candy, pastries, honey, and sucrose (table sugar)

→ Slow-acting sugar (or complex carbohydrate) containing starch, such as potatoes, peas, lentils, pasta, rice, and bread; these require several hours to be absorbed and act as true fuel

If you consume more carbohydrate than your body needs, it is stored as glycogen in the liver and muscles and as fat in the cells. If you eat too much carbohydrate, it means you are eating too many calories. This causes trouble with your metabolism and can lead to obesity, diabetes, digestive issues, and even dental cavities.

VITAMINS

Vitamins are necessary for the proper functioning of your body. They activate the transformation of foods and facilitate the use of energy.

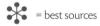 = best sources   ➡ = recommended amount for an adult

VITAMIN A is the growth vitamin.
Essential for sight, skin, hair, and strength of teeth and bones. It protects against infections in the mucous membranes in the lungs, the digestive tract, and urinary tract.

 Butter, milk, cheese, egg yolks, veal liver, fish, spinach, lettuce, carrots, apricots, melons, and all red fruits.

➡ 12 milligrams per day.

VITAMIN E is the anti-rickets and anti-aging vitamin.

 Butter, sunflower oil, olive oil, egg yolks, fatty fish, corn, wheat.

➡ 20 milligrams per day.

VITAMIN F lends elasticity to tissues and helps with proper intestinal function.

 Wheat germ and sunflower oil.

➡ 2 to 6 milligrams per day.

VITAMIN K is an excellent anti-hemorrhaging agent. It promotes blood clotting.

 Spinach, potatoes, fruits, cabbages, tomatoes, vegetable oils, liver, yogurt, egg yolks.

➡ 4 milligrams per day.

VITAMIN B₃ (niacin) is necessary for proper cell function. It prevents digestive troubles and dehydration of the skin.

 Salmon, tomatoes, nuts, wheat germ, veal.

➡ 15 milligrams per day.

VITAMINS B₁ AND B₂ are essential for the central nervous system and the cells. Vitamin B_1 governs the transformation of sugar and fat. Vitamin B_2 improves the skin. These two vitamins help increase the resistance to external attacks on your body, such as viruses, fatigue, and stress.

 B_1: Liver, pork, radishes, egg yolks, vegetables, dried fruits. B_2: Fish, cereal, prunes, mushrooms.

➡ 1 to 2 milligrams per day.

VITAMIN C is a true cure-all.
It helps fight fatigue, governs the assimilation of calcium, participates in skeletal growth, and stimulates the response of the immune system. It is because of this vitamin that the suprarenal and adrenal glands synthesize hormones in response to stress. It strengthens teeth, gums, ligaments, and blood vessels and promotes scarring.

 Citrus fruits, apples, pears, kiwis, strawberries, grapes, and all fresh vegetables, salads, broccoli, cabbages, watercress, and parsley. Red peppers are very rich in vitamin C.

➡ 70 milligrams per day.

VITAMIN D fixes calcium in the bones. Its role is therefore essential in the construction of the skeleton. It is excellent at fighting rickets.

Seafood, fish, butter, milk, egg yolks.

➡ 1 to 2 milligrams per day.

MINERALS AND TRACE ELEMENTS

Minerals and trace elements, even in tiny quantities, are essential for balancing your metabolism. Each is involved in chemical reactions in the body, yet they represent only 1 percent of the mass of the human body. They are primarily found in foods and mineral water. A deficiency in a single trace element can put your energy balance in peril by causing your body to revert to other energy sources. Then you risk suffering extreme fatigue, sudden tired spells, or a drop in blood pressure.

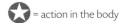 = action in the body   = best sources

 = secondary effects and toxicity

➡ = recommended amount for an adult

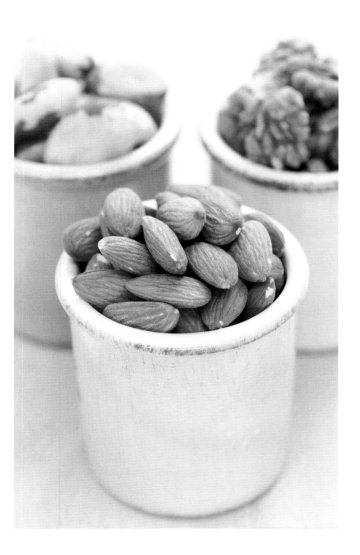

PHOSPHORUS is involved in construction of the skeleton.

⭐	Metabolism of carbohydrate, protein, fat; growth, repair and maintenance of tissues; and production of energy. It's involved in muscle contraction.
✳	Dairy products, Gruyère cheese, egg yolks, rice, lentils, soy, dried beans, almonds, nuts, meats, fish, poultry, eggs, whole grains, plant oils.
⊗	None known.
➡	1,000 to 3,000 milligrams per day.

POTASSIUM helps regulate blood pressure by intervening chemically between protein and carbohydrate. This metal, widely available in salt form, plays an important role in electrolyte balance in the body.

⭐	Maintenance of proper water balance on each side of the cell, promotes normal growth, transmits nerve impulses initiating muscle contraction, participates in the conversion of glucose into glycogen and in the synthesis of muscle proteins from amino acids.
✳	Potatoes, chocolate, bananas, fruits, green vegetables.
⊗	Heart problems.
➡	2.5 to 3.5 milligrams per day.

CALCIUM provides strength in the bones and teeth (where 99 percent of it is located). It also plays a part in the permeability of cell membranes and is involved in several steps of blood coagulation. It protects ligaments and joints and participates in contraction of nerve impulses.

⭐	Component of structures in the body; vital in growth and muscle contraction and in the transmission of nerve impulses.
✳	All mineral waters and dairy products (only sources of absorbable calcium): milk, yogurt, cottage cheese, cheese.
⊗	Excessive calcification of certain tissues, constipation, problems absorbing other minerals.
➡	1,000 milligrams per day.

CHROMIUM ensures the stability of sugar and fat in metabolism. It is necessary for proper balance even though you need to consume only tiny amounts of it; otherwise it can be toxic.

 Ensures sugar and fat are metabolized normally.

Brewer's yeast, corn oil, whole grains, liver, meats.

⊗ Kidney and liver problems.

➡ 2 to 3 milligrams per day.

SODIUM is an element that predominates in the blood and in extracellular liquids of the body. It is essential for maintaining the balance of water in the body as well as in regulating blood pressure.

 Maintains proper water balance on each side of the cell, contracts muscle, transmits nerve impulses, permits the solubility of other ions in the blood.

Is found in all foods.

⊗ Water retention and high blood pressure.

➡ 5 milligrams per day.

IODINE is excellent for vision and the skin.

 Production of energy, growth and development, and metabolism. Essential for balance in the thyroid gland.

Seafood and mushrooms. The regular consumption of iodized salt is sufficient to cover your body's needs.

⊗ Increase in size of the thyroid gland.

➡ 100 milligrams per day.

MAGNESIUM is a muscle relaxant. It promotes the transmission of nerve impulses (bundles of filaments from a group of neurons that go toward the same anatomical region), revitalizes the cells, and protects heart tissue.

 Metabolism of carbohydrate and protein, neuromuscular contractions.

 Dried vegetables, seafood, cocoa, dried fruits, certain mineral waters, whole grains, wheat germ, Swiss chard, pastries, almonds, rolled oats.

⊗ Toxic at high doses.

➡ 400 milligrams per day for men.
350 milligrams per day for women.

IRON is indispensable for manufacturing hemoglobin.*
It increases muscle work and acts on heart muscle. It also promotes the elimination of toxins. The lack of iron in the body results in fatigue, vertigo, and anemia.

 Transports oxygen to tissues to provide energy and formation of red blood cells to transport oxygen.

Liver, blood sausage, oysters, lean meats, seafood, giblets, beef, eggs, green vegetables, spinach, parsley, wheat, soy.

⊗ Toxic and an oxidizer at high doses. Can cause digestive problems. Harmful to the liver, pancreas, and cardiac activity.

➡ 12 milligrams per day.

* Protein pigments in red blood cells that carry oxygen in the blood.

ZINC is essential for growth and proper organ development.

 Excellent for scarring of wounds and burns. Regulates the activity of protein and hormones. Indispensable for growth, reproduction, and the nervous system.

Shellfish (especially oysters), fish, dried vegetables, green vegetables, veal, turkey, wheat germ, whole grains, nuts, hazelnuts, soy, veal and sheep liver; fructose helps its assimilation.

⊗ At high doses, deficits of copper and high blood cholesterol have been observed.

➡ 10 to 15 milligrams per day.

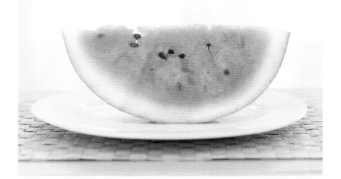

HOW TO WORK YOUR BUTTOCKS AND ABDOMINAL MUSCLES

Working the buttocks and abdominal muscles will help you sculpt a beautiful silhouette and shed unsightly fat. Before you begin your training program, here is what you need to know to obtain the results you desire.

SCULPT YOUR BUTT

Aesthetically, the buttocks certainly have a unique role. Well-rounded buttocks attract attention. Through targeted work, your goal is to shape them and improve their contour.

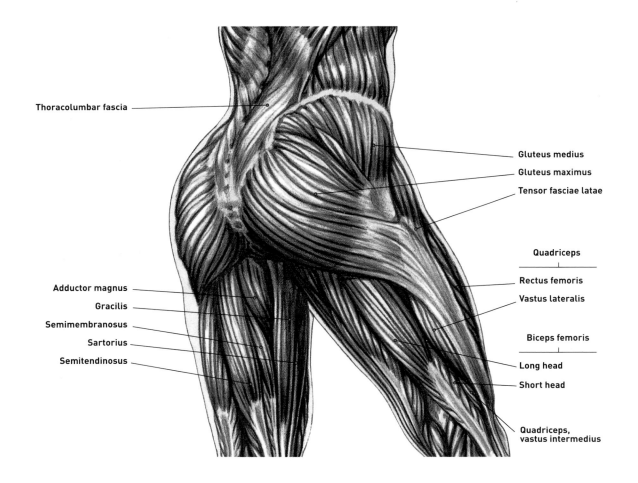

Thoracolumbar fascia

Gluteus medius

Gluteus maximus

Tensor fasciae latae

Quadriceps

Rectus femoris

Vastus lateralis

Biceps femoris

Adductor magnus

Gracilis

Semimembranosus

Sartorius

Semitendinosus

Long head

Short head

Quadriceps, vastus intermedius

ANATOMICAL CONSIDERATIONS

The buttocks are made up of several muscles. Each has a specific function and influences your curves.

→ The gluteus maximus is the largest and most powerful muscle in the human body. It makes up most of the buttocks. When it is toned, it gives a rounded aspect to the buttocks.

→ The gluteus medius is an abductor situated laterally. When it is muscular, it firms the upper buttocks and creates an appealing curve, making the small of the back beautiful. It allows the extension of the hip during lateral raise exercises.

→ The gluteus minimus is also an abductor situated deeply below the gluteus medius. This is the muscle that, when it is not firm, forms fat reserves commonly called saddlebags.

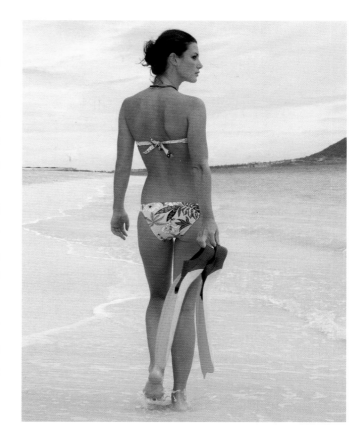

ROLE OF THE BUTTOCKS MUSCLES

The butt is made up of a large amount of fat and muscles, together called the buttocks. The buttocks support the muscles of the thighs, called the hamstrings, when you need to increase your running speed. Thus, when you walk slowly, they work very little, but as soon as you speed up, they begin to work.

TIPS FOR A MORE EFFECTIVE WORKOUT

→ If you desire toned buttocks, then you need to perform regular physical activity and eat a balanced diet. In fact, to increase the effectiveness of localized muscle development, exercise must be combined with an ideal diet. It is also recommended that you do firming exercises, preferably before meals.

→ To increase the effectiveness of the exercises, squeeze your buttocks as tightly as you can throughout the exercises. At first, you might have trouble doing this. But after several sessions, this reflex will become automatic if you are really concentrating.

→ If you do not have a lot of fat to lose, know that these exercises can be done preventively. In fact, fat typically accumulates above muscles that are not used often in daily life. The butt and the abdominal muscles rarely work; this is why fat often accumulates in these areas.

Importance of a Warm-Up

Warming up is an essential step before doing any physical exercise.

Before exercise, a warm-up will ensure that your body functions properly. It allows you to make your muscles and joints more flexible. It also protects you from potential injuries by preventing trauma to your joints and tendons. It also lets the blood vessels in your heart have an ample supply of oxygen before exercise. In this way, your heart will be prepared for either a brief or prolonged physical effort. You need to warm up progressively for only 5 to 10 minutes to prepare your joints, increase your flexibility, and begin cardiorespiratory work. A warm-up raises your body temperature. This heat makes the synovial fluid (a natural lubricant found in your joints) warmer and thereby improves the range of motion of your joints. The heat increases the resistance of your muscles, while cold has the opposite effect. Finally, a good warm-up improves your mental outlook because you feel better and more focused when your body is warm than when it is cold.

Skipping a warm-up will cause you to have pain later and a diminished capacity to train effectively. Furthermore, if you warm up, your body will feel more comfortable and flexible, and your concentration will only improve.

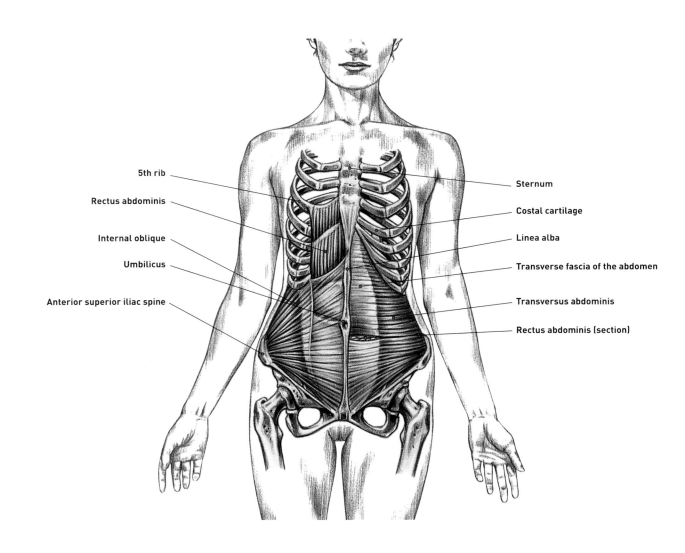

5th rib

Rectus abdominis

Internal oblique

Umbilicus

Anterior superior iliac spine

Sternum

Costal cartilage

Linea alba

Transverse fascia of the abdomen

Transversus abdominis

Rectus abdominis (section)

SCULPT YOUR ABS

The core and abdominal muscles play an important role in the body's aesthetics. Getting a muscular and toned belly in a few months is possible with targeted exercises. Say good-bye to your love handles and belly!

ANATOMICAL CONSIDERATIONS

The abdominal wall is made up of four muscles:

1. The rectus abdominis is usually called the abs.
2. The external oblique is located on either side of the rectus abdominis.
3. The internal oblique is located underneath the external oblique.
4. The transversus abdominis is located under the obliques.

Unlike other muscles where you want to develop some size, here the focus is on keeping the waist small by having well-defined muscles.

....

Muscles in a Slim Waist

....

The rectus abdominis does help contain the belly, but there are some less well-known muscles that make the waist as small as possible:

→ *Transversus abdominis acts just like a corset.*
→ *Internal and external obliques, to a lesser degree, also help to refine the waist when they are toned but not too muscular.*

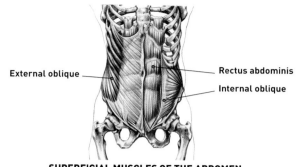

External oblique — Rectus abdominis
Internal oblique

SUPERFICIAL MUSCLES OF THE ABDOMEN

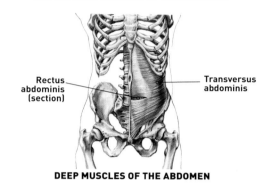

Rectus abdominis (section) — Transversus abdominis

DEEP MUSCLES OF THE ABDOMEN

ROLE OF THE ABDOMINAL MUSCLES

When talking about the abdominal muscles, the first thing that comes to mind is definitely looks: Well-defined abs are synonymous with a flat belly void of any extra fat. But Mother Nature did not give you abdominal muscles just to look nice. The abdominal wall fulfills vital functions for movement and health. There are six good reasons to take care of your abdominal wall:

1. Increase your athletic performance. The core plays a large role in all physical activities requiring rapid running or twisting of the torso (such as golf or tennis).

2. Protect your spine. In concert with the lumbar muscles, the abdominal muscles support the spine. Weak core and abdominal muscles and a large belly increase the risk of lumbar degeneration.

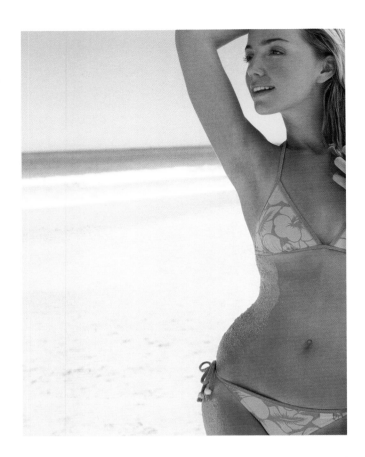

the upper part. It is possible to do bridges primarily using the strength of the upper abdominal muscles. However, the lower abdominal muscles play the most important role in protecting the spine and preventing bloating in the abdomen. And it is also this part that tends to accumulate fat most easily. A good training program should therefore work both the upper and lower parts of the abdominal muscles. You should know that exercises that involve raising the torso recruit mostly (but not exclusively) the upper part of the abdominal muscles. Exercises that involve lifting the pelvis target the lower part a little better.

TIPS FOR A MORE EFFECTIVE WORKOUT

→ It is important to breathe well during a set of abdominal and core exercises. The tendency is to hold your breath, but this is a mistake since breathing gives you more endurance by providing oxygen to your muscles during exercise.

→ Beware of fake abdominal exercises! Fake exercises, unfortunately, are very common. They are ineffective and put the spine in danger. There is a way to differentiate the good exercises from the bad. When the abdominal muscles contract, they round the lower back. So any exercise that arches the lumbar region instead of rounding your back cannot work the abdominal muscles effectively.

→ Beware of your head position! The position of your head has a profound impact on muscle contraction; when you lean your head back, the lumbar muscles that support the spine contract reflexively, while the abdominal muscles have a tendency to relax.

3. Reduce muscle tension. A few minutes of core and abs work before going to sleep will relax the lumbar muscles, allowing the spine to decompress from the pressure experienced during the day. No more waking up in the morning with back pain.

4. Improve digestive health. Core and abs work improves digestion of food, thereby preventing bloating and constipation.

5. Reduce risk factors for health conditions such as diabetes.

6. Maintain cardiovascular health. Working the core and abdominal muscles is an excellent cardiorespiratory workout, similar to running but without the trauma to the knees and the spine.

Unfortunately, the lower part of the abdominal muscles is much more difficult to strengthen than

Even if this contraction is not very strong, it is inevitable. On the contrary, when you lean your head forward, the abdominal muscles contract while the lumbar muscles relax; the body tends to round forward. The most common mistake is to look up at the ceiling, when you actually need to keep your head leaning forward and your back rounded. Ideally, you should always keep your eyes on your abs. What you must avoid above all is moving your head from side to side. This movement is not useful and can hamper proper muscle contraction. It also can cause cervical problems. In the same way, it is counterproductive to move your head frenetically when the exercise gets really difficult. Instead, your body must be very stable when an exercise gets difficult.

→ Take care in the placement of your hands and elbows during sit-ups. To avoid pulling too much on your neck, do not cross your hands behind your head; rather, place them on your ears. Note that the wider you place your elbows, the harder the exercise will be. Conversely, the closer your elbows are together and the more they tilt toward the front, the easier the exercise will be.

→ Do not confuse pulling your abdomen in with contracting your abdomen. When you have to pull on a pair of tight jeans, you suck in your abdomen by pulling the abdominal fibers up (without any particular tone) so you can fasten the button. However, abdominal contraction is a compression of the fibers that lets you strengthen and tone this part of the body. Do not forget that all your strength comes from your core and that this contraction stabilizes the body, providing support

and power. If you do abdominal work by pulling your abdomen in, you will have no chance at all of developing your abdominal muscles.

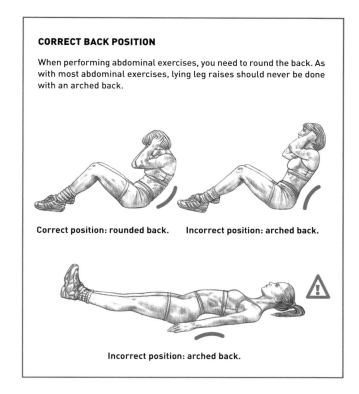

CORRECT BACK POSITION

When performing abdominal exercises, you need to round the back. As with most abdominal exercises, lying leg raises should never be done with an arched back.

Correct position: rounded back.   Incorrect position: arched back.

Incorrect position: arched back.

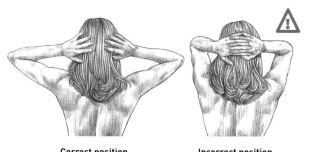

CORRECT PLACEMENT OF HANDS AND ELBOWS

So that you do not pull too hard on your neck, do not cross your hands behind your head; rather, place them on your ears. Note that the wider you place your elbows, the harder the exercise will be. Conversely, the closer your elbows are together and the more toward the front, the easier the exercise will be.

Correct position.   Incorrect position.

Posterior Pelvic Tilt

Imagine that your abdominal wall is a large belt going from your hips to your ribs. The width of the belt does not change, but you can tighten or loosen it.

Pulling in your abdomen and contracting your abdominal muscles are not the same thing, but this idea can help you recruit your abdominal muscles if you imagine that your navel is the buckle of the belt and that you are trying to pull it toward your spine to buckle the belt, but without moving your ribs. You do not hollow out your belly; you just recruit your muscle "belt" to form a corset that will protect the entire lumbar region, especially during abdominal exercises and certain buttocks exercises.

This intense recruitment of the abdominal muscles is accompanied by a contraction of the buttocks muscles, and the two create a natural movement of the pelvis toward the back that is called a posterior pelvic tilt. Try this test: Stand up straight, without contracting your abdominal or buttocks muscles. Your pelvis is in a neutral position. Now, arch your back and move your buttocks toward the back. You will definitely feel that when your pelvis is tilted toward the front, in an anterior tilt, it is difficult to recruit your muscles. Come back to a neutral position and tilt your pelvis backward: In a posterior tilt, you mobilize your abdominal and buttocks muscles naturally.

This position protects the spine and especially the lower back. It should be used as the starting position in some exercises in which it is important not to arch your back to avoid injury and to recruit the abdominal and buttocks muscles effectively.

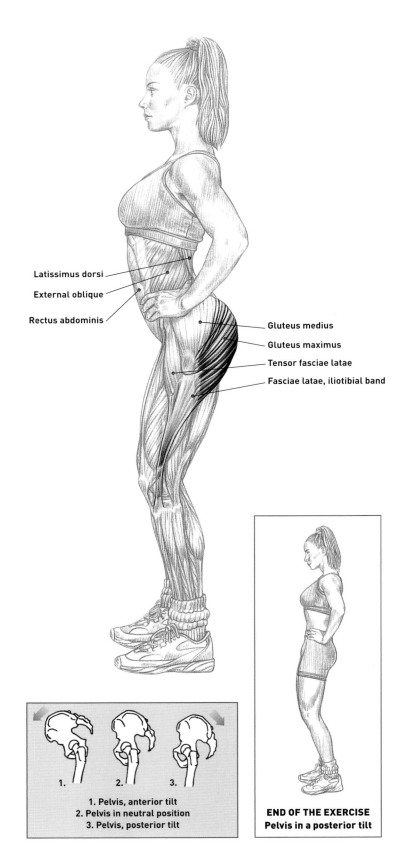

Latissimus dorsi
External oblique
Rectus abdominis
Gluteus medius
Gluteus maximus
Tensor fasciae latae
Fasciae latae, iliotibial band

1. Pelvis, anterior tilt
2. Pelvis in neutral position
3. Pelvis, posterior tilt

END OF THE EXERCISE
Pelvis in a posterior tilt

GET RID OF CELLULITE

Cellulite is a typically feminine phenomenon where subcutaneous fat accumulates in certain areas, primarily the lower part of the body. It is made up of a mixture of water, waste, and toxins in the skin tissue and fatty tissue in certain cells. Cellulite happens to two out of three women, including those who are not overweight.

TWO TYPES OF CELLULITE

The first kind of cellulite is characterized by a lack of suppleness and elasticity in the skin. When you pinch your skin between two fingers, it is puffy and looks like the skin of an orange. Though cellulite may not always reach the skin, it noticeably degrades it. It is rough and sometimes wrinkled, and the skin is dehydrated and a little warm. This kind of cellulite is unsightly, and it is visible no matter what position your body is in.

The second kind of cellulite is a little different: The skin tissue is spongy and flabby. The cellulite looks different depending on whether you are standing (it diminishes) or lying down (it spreads). There are often stretch marks on the skin where elasticity has been broken. This kind of cellulite mostly occurs in women over 35 years of age. It can also appear after losing a substantial amount of weight, from losing weight too quickly, and from taking too many diuretic supplements.

REASONS YOU GET CELLULITE

The appearance of cellulite depends on numerous factors such as a rich diet, a sedentary lifestyle, and poor blood circulation. Genetic factors must be taken into consideration as well as the influence of hormones (estrogen in particular). Before menstruation and during pregnancy, insufficient blood or lymphatic circulation and excess estrogen can encourage water retention.

Water Retention

When water carrying waste and residue accumulates and stagnates in porous pockets under the skin, it is called water retention. It happens during periods of stress or during a menstrual cycle and then goes away after a few days without any special treatment, except following a strict diet of no sugar and little salt. Cellulite occurs when this water becomes gelatinous, hardens, and creates pressure under the skin.

Only through an intense localized treatment of the fatty mass will you be able to dislodge this orange-peel skin texture, and this will tend to become more difficult over time.

HORMONAL CHANGES

The appearance and development of cellulite are linked to important hormonal stages in women's lives, such as puberty and pregnancy. Menopause is characterized by the ovaries' ceasing to function and produce hormones. You should know that at this stage of life, even though your body tends to activate fat cells less often, this does not mean you will not accumulate cellulite.

STRESS

Cellulite can occur during a period of intense prolonged stress and be linked to gynecological, circulatory, and digestive problems. These can seriously aggravate cellulite. In fact, the liver plays an essential role in digesting food. If digestion is not occurring properly, then liver function slows down. Fat and sugar will be stored, and your body will retain toxins that will considerably alter your skin tissue.

PRIMARY LOCATIONS FOR FAT STORAGE

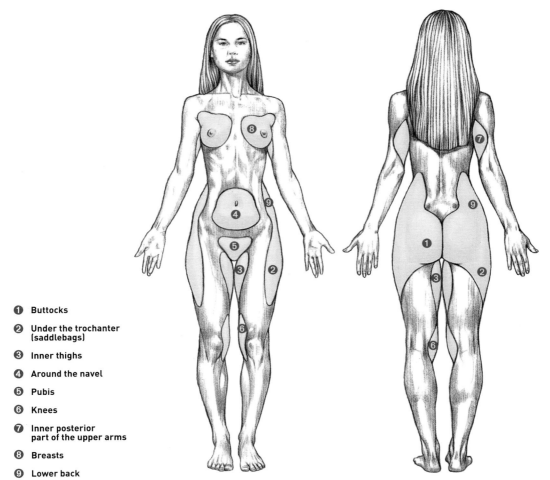

❶ Buttocks

❷ Under the trochanter (saddlebags)

❸ Inner thighs

❹ Around the navel

❺ Pubis

❻ Knees

❼ Inner posterior part of the upper arms

❽ Breasts

❾ Lower back

HEREDITY

Heredity seems to be an important factor in the development of cellulite, just as it is for obesity. (Women who have varicose veins and circulation problems often pass them on to their daughters).

You must be vigilant, though, because you are not doomed. By eating a diet low in sugar and by working your legs, you can break this hereditary chain.

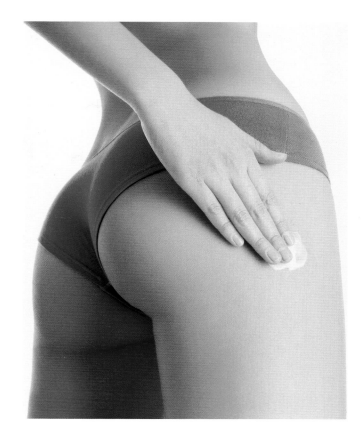

Cellulite on a Slim Physique

You can be thin and still have cellulite. In this case, there is no need for drastic dietary changes, but you should still take certain dietary precautions. To avoid accumulating fat in your tissues and replacing soft cellulite with hard, unmovable cellulite, you should eat a diet rich in protein and water and low in salt. And, of course, you should do some kind of sustained physical activity.

HOW TO BEAT CELLULITE

It is difficult to get rid of cellulite. You have to combine several methods, especially since it is resistant to weight loss.

ANTI-CELLULITE CREAMS

The major problem with diets is that they eliminate inches all over your body except in those problem areas where you really want to lose weight! Anti-cellulite creams are designed to be applied to those trouble spots. They contain molecules that mobilize fat (such as caffeine, aminophylline and theophylline, and forskolin), others that improve circulation (such as gotu kola, ruscogenin, and ginkgo biloba), and

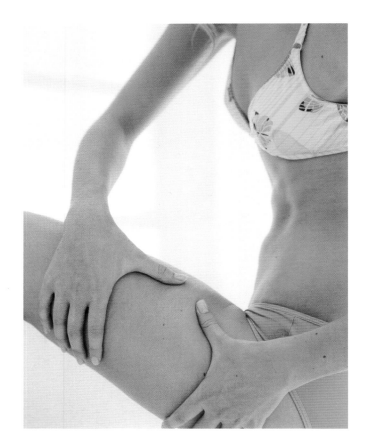

microcirculation and the removal of retained water and will reduce the ability of fat cells to grow. The virtues of massage outweigh any effectiveness of anti-cellulite creams.

PLASTIC SURGERY

In parallel with deep work on cellulite, you could enlist the help of a plastic surgeon. In cases where there is a large amount of cellulite, even intense physical activity will not completely solve the problem. A physician can perform an operation under local anesthesia. The doctor uses a tube attached to an aspirator to reach the fatty tissue and suck it out. But if you do not adopt a strict diet and exercise regularly after the operation, then all the cellulite will come back. And, of course, as with any surgery, there are risks involved.

MASSAGE

Once you have a diet in place that does not include snacking and fast sugar (such as cakes and candy) and you are regularly doing the exercises from this book, pay careful attention to your body. Get in the habit of massaging yourself to improve blood circulation in the mornings and evenings. Focus on the pads of fat and press them under your fingers. Roll them so that you can start to soften them. You can use some of the many massage creams on the market (effective only on superficial cellulite) that are primarily made to soften and hydrate the skin. You should have regular massages to promote lymphatic circulation and reduce water retention.

some that improve the skin's appearance (such as retinol and silicon). The effectiveness of these creams, however, is limited:

→ They work only on a superficial level. When you stop applying them, you gain the inches back quickly, which proves that this loss is the result of localized water loss rather than a true loss of fat.

→ Beyond acting on fat cells, regularly applying creams that hydrate, tighten, or thicken the skin will hide cellulite. The orange-peel skin will quickly return once you stop applying the cream. However, hydrating creams are significantly less expensive than anti-cellulite creams.

→ Whether the cream is active or not, regularly massaging areas that have cellulite will promote

Massaging the capillaries under the skin activates the lymphatic vessels that transport waste from cells into the blood, where they are removed.

INTENSE EXERCISES

If at first the weight loss generated by a diet seems to make cellulite more noticeable, with targeted and in-depth regular exercise, you can confine cellulite and stop it from expanding. Since cellulite is primarily located on the lower part of the body, the exercises will be focused on the lower part of the body as well.

At first, the exercises will help activate blood circulation through flexion movements (forward lunge); then they will work the thigh muscles and the knees by using sets that are longer and closer together. Increasing the sets and decreasing the recovery time are two conditions for burning fat. Here, breathing is key: Proper oxygenation will help you persevere in the exercise because the muscle will be better oxygenated during the exercise and can be worked in depth. Exercises that focus on eliminating cellulite are particularly difficult to sustain. You will not be able to do them correctly without deep, long breaths. Running is a great cardiorespiratory exercise that gets the blood moving. The same is true of stair machines, which have two steps that you press with your feet, alternating the right and left feet. It works your buttocks and thighs. Of course, any exercise that develops the buttocks will help get rid of saddlebags. Exercises using ankle weights will refine your knees, but here again, you will want to use long sets and short recovery times.

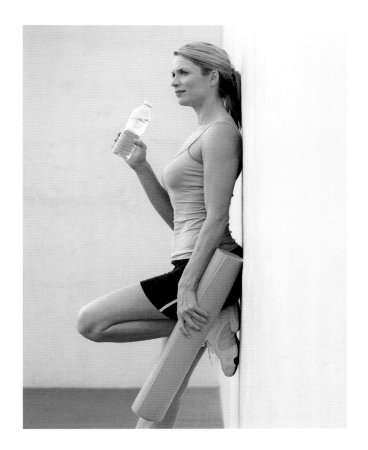

A Few Anti-Cellulite Tips

→ *You need to move to activate your blood circulation: Climb stairs and change positions frequently.*
→ *Drink a lot of water: 6 to 8 glasses each day.*
→ *Sleep with your legs elevated 6 inches (15 cm).*
→ *Do not smoke.*
→ *Do not wear clothes that fit too tightly.*
→ *Avoid exposure to heat, such as very hot baths and prolonged exposure to the sun.*
→ *To avoid putting pressure on circulatory vessels, do not cross your legs.*
→ *Give yourself massages.*
→ *Wear shoes with heels that are no more than 2 inches high (<5 cm) for better circulation in your veins.*

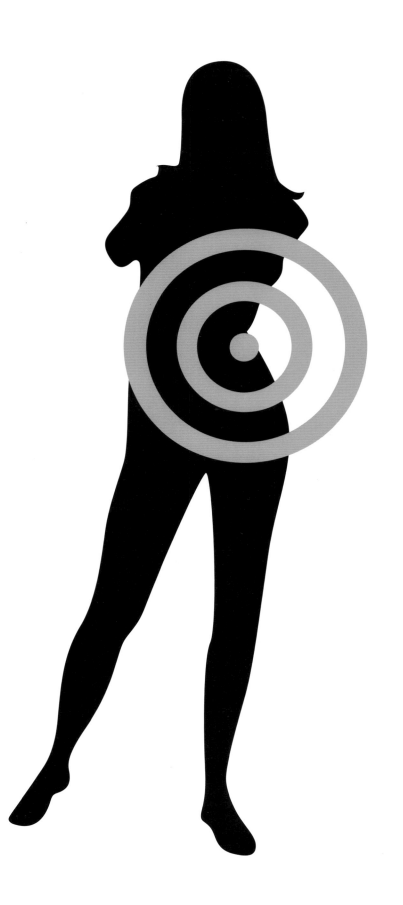

GOAL 1
Slim Your Waist

Static Stretch for the Waist

Targets   Stretches your waist while reducing pressure and tension in your spinal joints.

Repetitions   Hold the stretch for 20 to 30 seconds and repeat 3 or 4 times.

Your coach's advice   Concentrate on pulling in your abdomen and tightening your buttocks during this stretch.

Breathing   Inhale and exhale deeply while you hold the stretch.

Warning   When doing the variation where you lean your torso to the side, you can bend your knees slightly to relieve pressure on your lumbar spine.

Key to the exercise   Tighten your abdominal wall, but be very careful not to hold your breath!

1. Stand with your legs apart and your feet parallel. Tighten your buttocks and your abdominal muscles. Interlace your fingers and straighten your arms above your head while turning your hands to the outside.

2. Inhale so that you can inflate your chest and stretch your ribs (intercostal muscles). Push your hands up high while keeping your head and back very straight.

3. Exhale slowly as you relax. Repeat the stretch.

★ **Variation**   If you lean your torso to the side and hold the stretch for 20 to 30 seconds on the right side and then on the left side, you will stretch both the internal and external obliques as well as the quadratus lumborum more intensely. You must be careful not to move your hips when you lower your torso or when you come back up.

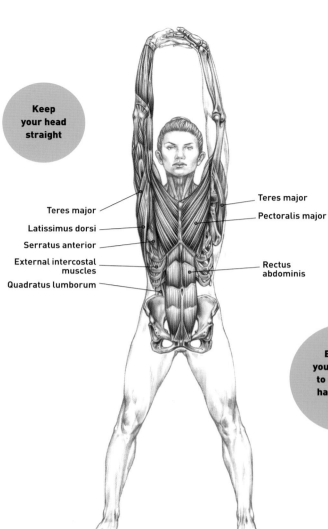

Keep your head straight

Teres major

Latissimus dorsi

Serratus anterior

External intercostal muscles

Quadratus lumborum

Teres major

Pectoralis major

Rectus abdominis

Each time you exhale, try to reach your hands a little higher

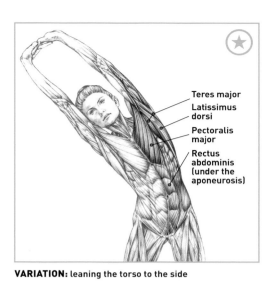

Teres major

Latissimus dorsi

Pectoralis major

Rectus abdominis (under the aponeurosis)

VARIATION: leaning the torso to the side

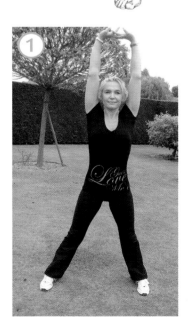

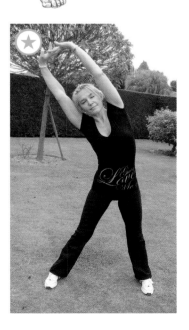

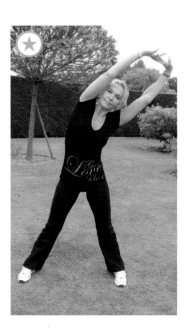

Standing Side Bend

Targets Stretches the waist while toning it. This exercise primarily works the obliques to help slim the waist, but it also works the rectus abdominis muscle and the deep muscles of the back.

Repetitions Do 2 or 3 sets of 30 repetitions on each side.

Your coach's advice In this exercise, you must disassociate your lower body from your upper body. During the exercise, don't move your pelvis; otherwise you could engage your lumbar region. Only the upper part of your body moves, and you can really work your waist.

Breathing Exhale as you lower your torso and inhale as you come up. You could also inhale throughout one repetition (lowering and raising the torso) and exhale during the next repetition.

Warning It is better not to go down as low and keep your pelvis very stable than to go down too far and end up moving your hips.

Key to the exercise Turn your feet out to help with your balance and so that you can contract your buttocks even more (this will also keep you from compensating with your hips). Pull in your abdomen to stabilize your pelvis.

1. Stand with your feet shoulder-width apart and one hand behind your head. Grab a dumbbell with the other hand.

2. Exhale as you lean your torso to the side opposite the hand with the weight and keep your torso very straight.

3. Return to the starting position as you inhale, all while keeping your pelvis very still.

Variation You can do this exercise with a stick. The exercise will be easier and it will also be easier to keep your pelvis stable since this variation is done with the feet farther apart. You will also stretch the side of your torso more (serratus anterior and latissimus dorsi muscles). With a stick, you can bend your torso from side to side in a combination move. When using a dumbbell, you have to do a set on one side and then switch to the other side.

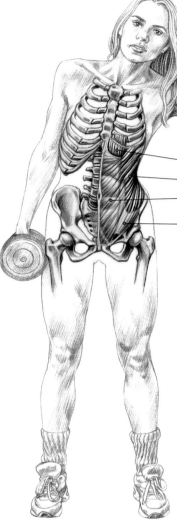

Keep your head straight

Rectus abdominis

External oblique

Rectus abdominis (under the aponeurosis)

Internal oblique (under the aponeurosis)

Do not move your pelvis to the side

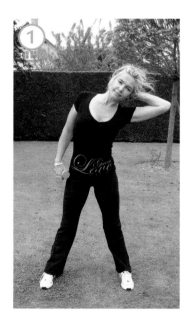

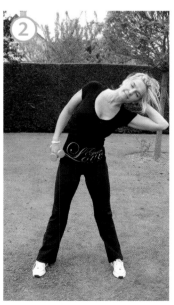

VARIATION: using a stick

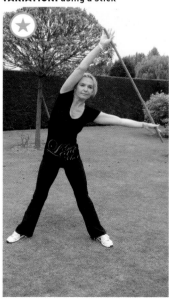

Torso Twist With a Stick

Targets   Tones the waist.

Repetitions   Do 3 or 4 sets of 30 repetitions on each side.

Your coach's advice   To avoid engaging your lower back too much, think about tilting your pelvis backward (see page 30). You can also bend your knees slightly if it helps to stabilize your pelvis. This position will also be easier on your joints.

Breathing   Exhale as you rotate your torso to the outside and inhale as you come back. You can also inhale throughout one repetition (rotation and return to the starting position) and exhale during the following repetition.

Warning   Contract your abdominal muscles and breathe correctly throughout the exercise. People who have lower back problems or who have had a herniated disc should not do torso twists since this exercise could aggravate or cause a recurrence of the problem.

Key to the exercise   To isolate your back muscles and waist, avoid moving your hips. For better stability, you can keep your legs a little bit wider than hip width.

1. Stand with your torso straight, legs apart, and feet slightly turned out for better stability. Grab a stick and rest it on your shoulder blades to keep from contracting your trapezius muscles (your hands should rest on the stick without pressing down).

2. Exhale as you twist your torso to the right. Inhale as you return to the starting position. Contract your buttocks muscles so that your pelvis faces forward throughout the exercise.

3. Perform the same rotation toward the left and then return to the starting position.

⭐ **Variation**   You can do this exercise while seated on a bench. This will help immobilize your pelvis so that you can better focus your efforts on the abdominal wall.

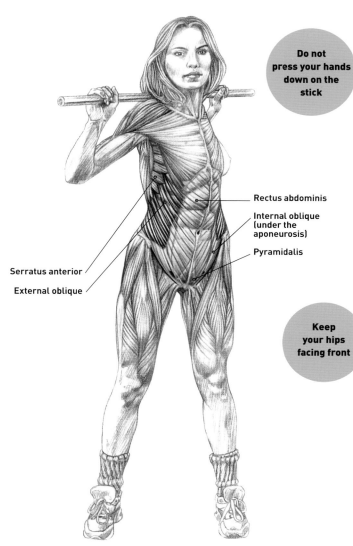

Do not press your hands down on the stick

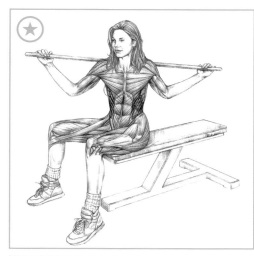

VARIATION: seated on a bench

Rectus abdominis

Internal oblique (under the aponeurosis)

Pyramidalis

Serratus anterior

External oblique

Keep your hips facing front

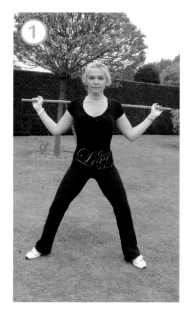

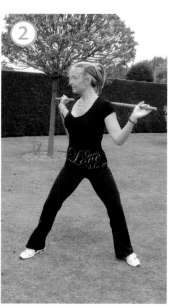

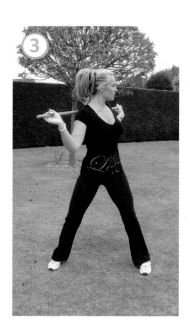

Lying Torso Twist

Targets Stretches and relaxes the back muscles.

Repetitions To relieve tension and relax your back muscles, do this exercise 1 or 2 times on each side and hold the stretch for about 30 to 40 seconds. To work and tone the waist, do 2 or 3 sets of 20 to 30 repetitions (alternating sides) without resting your knees on the floor.

Your coach's advice Lower your knees gently as you contract your abdominal muscles.

Breathing Inhale as you raise your knees and exhale as you lower them. If you are doing this as a static stretch, breathe regularly and constantly throughout the movement.

Warning Squeeze your knees together tightly and contract your abdominal muscles to avoid engaging your lumbar spine. Do not do this exercise if you have serious back problems.

Key to the exercise Be sure to keep your head and shoulders touching the floor so that you can really stretch your oblique muscles each time you lower your knees.

1 Lie on the floor with your arms straight out at the sides of your body and your palms on the floor. Keep your head in line with your body, and bend your knees.

2 Slowly let your knees fall to one side as you gently turn your head in the opposite direction. Let your knees go down as far as they can.

3 Hold this position for a few seconds to stretch your lower back or bring your knees back up as you inhale, depending on your goals.

★ **Variation** You can do this exercise with straight legs if you have very flexible hamstrings. But if this exercise seems a little difficult with your knees bent at a right angle, you can bring your knees closer to your chest.

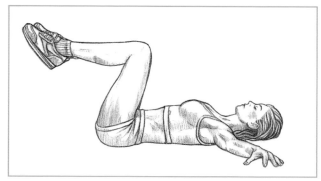

STARTING POSITION

Quadriceps femoris
Vastus medius
Vastus lateralis
Rectus femoris

Tensor fasciae latae

External oblique

Pectoralis major

Serratus anterior

Latissimus dorsi

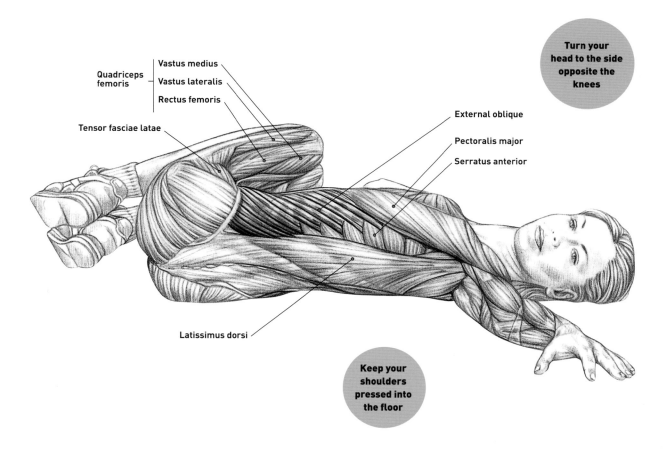

Turn your head to the side opposite the knees

Keep your shoulders pressed into the floor

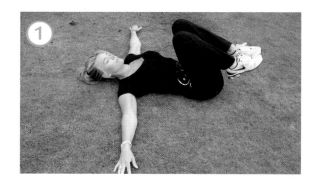

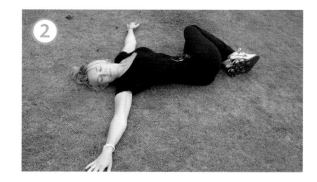

Side Plank

Targets   Works the serratus muscles and the external obliques to improve posture and the carriage of your head.

Repetitions   As a static stretch, hold the stretch for 10 to 30 seconds and repeat 3 times on each side. As a ballistic stretch, do 3 sets of 30 repetitions on each side.

Your coach's advice   Focus on tightening your abdominal and buttocks muscles so that you do not compensate with your back.

Breathing   Exhale as you raise your torso and then inhale as you lower your torso. In the static stretch, be sure that your breathing is even, slow, and deep.

Warning   The shoulders should be held down and away from the ears. If your form starts to deteriorate, you could injure yourself. It is better to focus on proper form over a shorter time.

Key to the exercise   Never rest your torso on the floor during this exercise; your hips should not touch the floor. This exercise works all the muscles responsible for good posture; that is why it will help you slim your waist and improve your posture.

1. Lie on your side with your arm bent to 90 degrees, your forearm resting on the floor, your shoulder directly above your elbow, and your other hand placed on your hip or upper thigh. Both of your legs should be straight and stacked on top of one another. Tighten your buttocks and abdominal muscles.

2. Exhale and lift your torso as high as you can. Your head, pelvis, and feet should form a line.

3. Inhale and slowly lower toward the floor. Then repeat until you complete your set.

Variation   You can also do this exercise statically by holding the raised position for 10 to 30 seconds. For horizontal stabilization, do the exercise statically as a front plank with both forearms resting on the floor. Be sure to keep your head in line with your spine and do not arch your back.

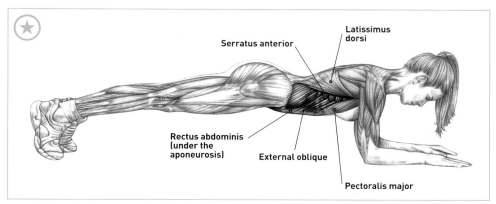

Latissimus dorsi

Rectus abdominis (under the aponeurosis)

External oblique

Pectoralis major

VARIATION: for horizontal stabilization

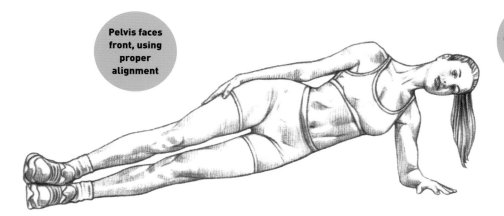

Pelvis faces front, using proper alignment

Shoulders down and away from the ears

Keep the head in line with the spine

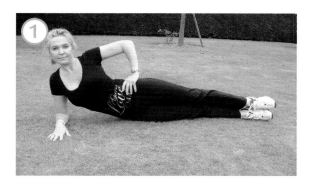

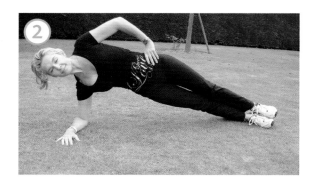

VARIATION: for horizontal stabilization

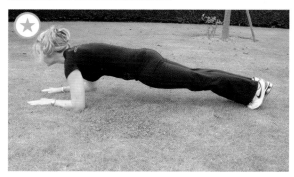

Swimming

Targets A very complete exercise that works the erector spinae muscles (lower back and lumbar region), the buttocks, and the muscles at the back of the shoulders.

Repetitions Do 3 or 4 sets of 15 to 20 repetitions. When doing the exercise statically, hold the position for 10 to 30 seconds and repeat 3 times.

Your coach's advice To avoid compensating with your lumbar muscles, think carefully about contracting your buttocks muscles (the navel is lifted slightly off the ground and pulled in toward the spine). Do not hold your breath.

Breathing Exhale as you stretch your arms in front of you and inhale as you bring them back behind you. When doing the exercise statically, be sure that your breathing is slow, deep, and even.

Warning Do not lift your head too high or you risk pinching your cervical spine. Do not lift your arms so high that you pull on your lumbar spine. If you have shoulder problems, you should do only the static variation of this exercise.

Key to the exercise Work your posture muscles: Mobilize the pelvic floor and contract the sphincter. This will give you more strength when performing the exercise, prevent injuries, and reinforce the effects of this exercise.

1. Lie on your belly on the floor with your arms in front of you and your legs straight behind you. Then inhale and, as you exhale, raise your feet and knees off the floor as well as your upper torso and arms.

2. Inhale and, as you exhale, raise your arms and legs a little higher, being careful to keep your head in line with your body.

3. On your next inhalation, bring your hands behind you in a breaststroke motion. Bring them above your buttocks but do not rest them on your buttocks. Exhale as you return to the starting position, and continue the swimming motion until the end of your set.

Variation You can do this exercise statically by holding your arms in front of you. In this case, hold the position for 10 to 30 seconds and, each time you exhale, try to raise your arms and legs a little higher. Be sure not to hurt your neck or arch your back.

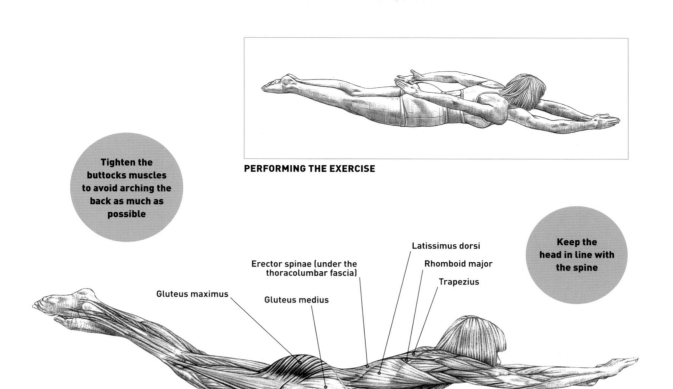

PERFORMING THE EXERCISE

Tighten the buttocks muscles to avoid arching the back as much as possible

Keep the head in line with the spine

Latissimus dorsi

Rhomboid major

Erector spinae (under the thoracolumbar fascia)

Trapezius

Gluteus maximus

Gluteus medius

External oblique

Serratus anterior

Shoulders down and away from the ears

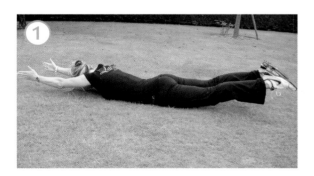

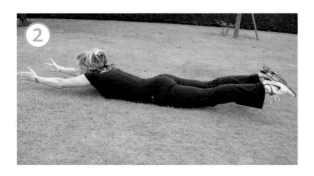

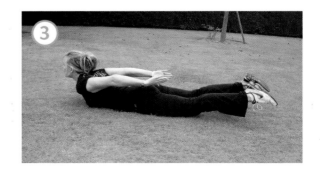

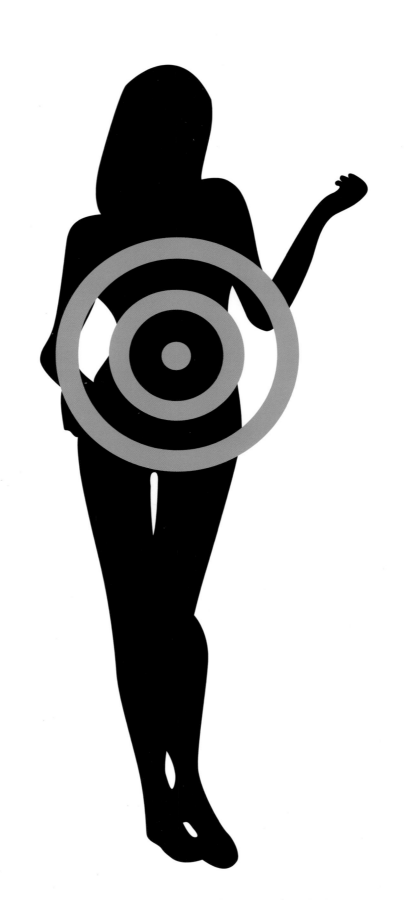

GOAL 2
Strengthen Your Abdominals

Crunch, Feet on the Floor

Targets　Works the rectus abdominis (upper abdominal muscle).

Repetitions　Do 4 sets of 20 to 30 repetitions.

Your coach's advice　Focus on pressing your back into the floor and contracting your abdominal muscles tightly. The abdominal muscles should be working, and you should not be compensating with your lower back. That said, unlike sit-ups, crunches have few risks; even people with back problems can do them.

Breathing　Exhale as you raise your torso and inhale as you lower it.

Warning　Do not place your hands behind your neck because you will end up pulling on your cervical vertebrae. Instead, place one hand near each ear.

Key to the exercise　The farther apart you hold your elbows, the harder the exercise will be. If you are a beginner, bring your elbows closer together and point them forward to make the exercise easier.

(1) Lie on the floor. Bend your legs and place your feet flat on the floor. Press your back into the floor and put your hands behind your head without interlacing your fingers.

(2) As you exhale, lift your head as much as you can and pull your upper back off of the floor, if you can. You should be looking at your navel.

(3) As you inhale, lower to the starting position, but do not rest your head on the floor. Take your time, and do 20 to 30 repetitions in this way.

Variation　You can also do this exercise with your legs resting on a bench (see pages 58-59) or with your legs held at 90 degrees. You can find this more difficult variation on the following pages.

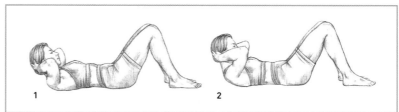

1. Starting position; 2. Performing the exercise

Look at your navel during the exercise

External oblique

Rectus abdominis (under the aponeurosis)

Place one hand on either side of your head

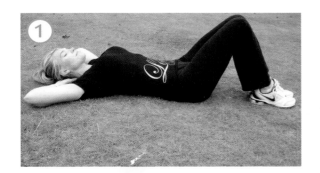

Rib

External intercostal muscle

Press your back into the floor

Lumbar vertebra

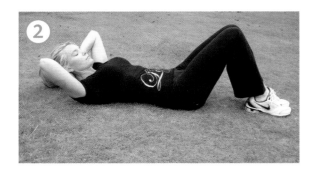

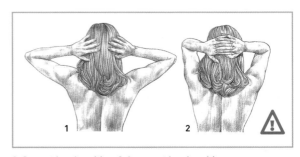

1. Correct hand position; 2. Incorrect hand position

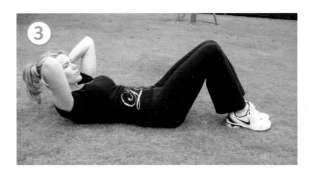

53

Crunch, Legs Raised

Targets　Works the rectus abdominis (upper abdominal muscle).

Repetitions　Do 4 sets of 20 to 30 repetitions.

Your coach's advice　As for all exercises that work the abdominal wall, simply looking at your navel by bringing your chin toward your chest creates a slight reflex contraction in the rectus abdominis muscle.

Breathing　Exhale as you raise your torso and inhale as you lower your torso.

Warning　Be careful where you place your hands. Press your back firmly into the floor.

Key to the exercise　Raising your legs and having your thighs in a vertical position will help you keep your lumbar spine pressed into the floor throughout the exercise. This way, you can really concentrate on your abdominal work. You can also cross your ankles if it helps you keep your legs steady. Your legs will stay in the same position throughout the exercise.

1. Lie with your back pressed into the floor and your hands behind your head without interlacing your fingers. Lift your legs so that your thighs are vertical and bend your knees 90 degrees.

2. As you exhale, slowly raise your head as much as you can and peel your upper back off the floor. Keep looking at your navel.

3. Inhale and lower to the starting position, but do not rest your head on the floor. Take your time, and do 20 to 30 repetitions in the same way.

★ **Variation**　You can also keep one leg bent with the foot flat on the floor and put your other foot on your thigh. As you exhale, roll up your spine to bring your head toward your knee or bring your knee toward your chest by lifting your foot off the floor. The first variation will work your upper abdominal muscles more, while the second variation will work the middle and lower abdominal muscles more.

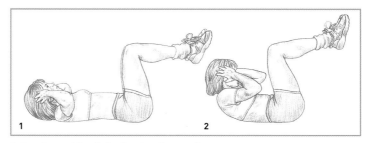

1. Starting position; 2. Performing the exercise

Look at your navel during the exercise

Abdominal muscle, upper part

Abdominal muscle, middle part

Abdominal muscle, lower part

Place one hand on either side of your head

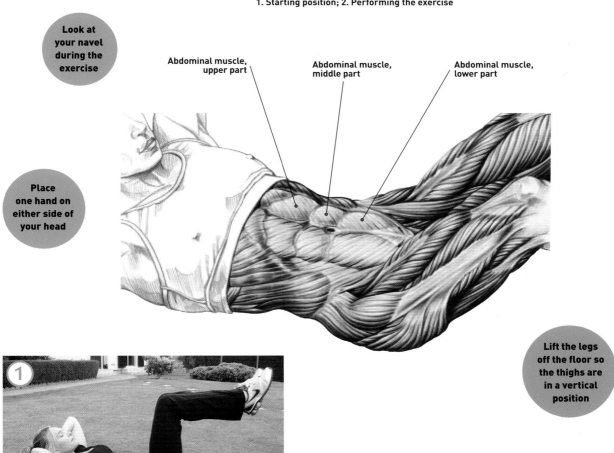

Lift the legs off the floor so the thighs are in a vertical position

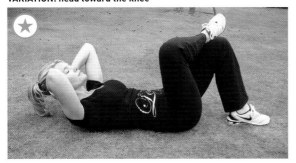

VARIATION: head toward the knee

VARIATION: knee toward the chest

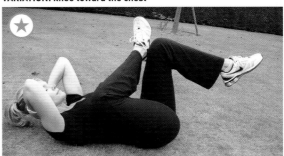

Sit-Up, Feet on the Floor

Targets   Works the rectus abdominis (upper abdominal muscle), but it also works the hip flexors as well as the internal and external obliques.

Repetitions   Do 4 sets of 20 to 30 repetitions.

Your coach's advice   Do your repetitions slowly in long sets. At the end of each set, you should feel a burning sensation in your abdomen. This means that the exercise is effective.

Breathing   Exhale as you go up and inhale as you go down.

Warning   Focus on contracting your abdominal muscles so that you do not engage the lumbar region. Keep your head in line with your body to avoid pulling on your cervical spine. Pay attention to the position of your hands if you are putting them behind your head.

Key to the exercise   It is important to round your back slightly throughout the exercise so that you can really feel your abdominal wall working. To work your abdominal wall even more intensely, you can lower your torso down halfway and then hold that position for 12 seconds before you come back up.

1. Lie on the floor with bent legs and feet flat on the floor. Press your back into the floor and put your arms alongside your body.

2. Exhale and raise your torso gradually without arching your back. Squeeze your abdominal muscles and keep your feet firmly on the floor. Your arms should be straight in front of you.

3. Inhale as you lower to the starting position, but do not rest your torso on the floor. Keep your feet and knees pressed together and do 20 to 30 repetitions in this way.

Variation   If you have difficulty keeping your feet on the floor, you can ask a partner to hold your feet for you or you can tuck them under a piece of furniture (such as a bed or sofa). Holding your arms out in front of you makes this exercise easier, so if you want a more difficult variation, put your hands behind your head. Just be careful not to interlace your fingers to avoid pulling on your cervical spine.

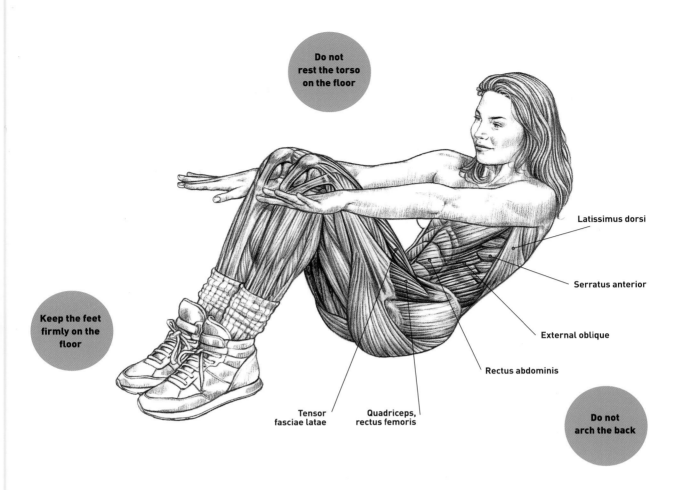

Do not rest the torso on the floor

Keep the feet firmly on the floor

Do not arch the back

Latissimus dorsi

Serratus anterior

External oblique

Rectus abdominis

Tensor fasciae latae

Quadriceps, rectus femoris

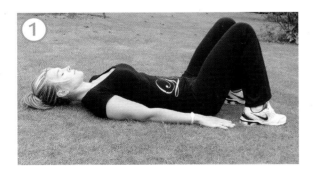

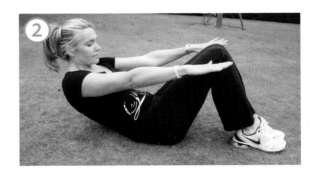

VARIATION: hands behind the head

VARIATION: feet held by a partner

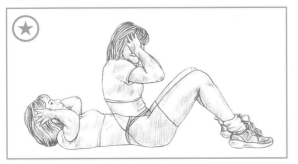

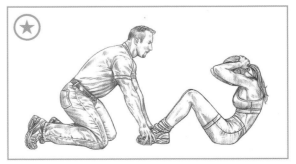

Crunch, Feet on a Bench

Targets   Works the rectus abdominis (upper abdominal muscle). The farther away your torso is from the bench, the more the tensor fasciae latae and the rectus femoris (front upper part of the thigh) will also work.

Repetitions   Do 3 or 4 sets of 20 to 30 repetitions.

Your coach's advice   Contract your abdominal muscles, "glue" your navel to your spine, and roll up your spine around this central point. Pay attention to the sensations in your body: You will notice that it is really the abdominal wall that is working and not other parts of the body compensating, causing you to cheat.

Breathing   Exhale as you raise your torso and inhale as you lower it.

Warning   So long as you roll up your back and do not just lift your torso, there is little risk of injury. Placing your legs on a bench will help you disassociate your upper body from your lower body, which will help you stabilize your pelvis. Still, you have to pay attention to the position of your hands to protect your cervical spine.

Key to the exercise   Do not rest your head on the floor. Always keep your head and shoulders slightly off the floor.

1. Lie on your back with bent legs, feet resting on a bench, and your back pressed firmly into the floor. Place your hands behind your head without interlacing your fingers.

2. As you exhale, contract your abdominal muscles and gradually raise your head as high as possible while lifting your upper back. Your lower back should remain on the floor.

3. As you inhale, lower to the starting position without resting your head on the floor. Do 20 to 30 repetitions slowly in this way, breathing deeply throughout.

Variation   If you are a beginner, stretch your arms in front of you and bring them toward your knees as you raise your torso. To focus the work on the upper part of the abdominal muscles, you can also hold your arms straight up toward the ceiling. Be gentle with your neck. When you do this variation, the range of motion will be smaller.

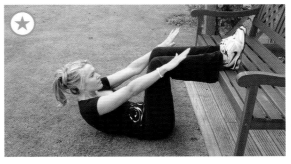

PERFORMING THE EXERCISE

Move the torso farther away from the bench to engage the upper thighs

Place one hand on either side of the head

Do not rest the head on the floor

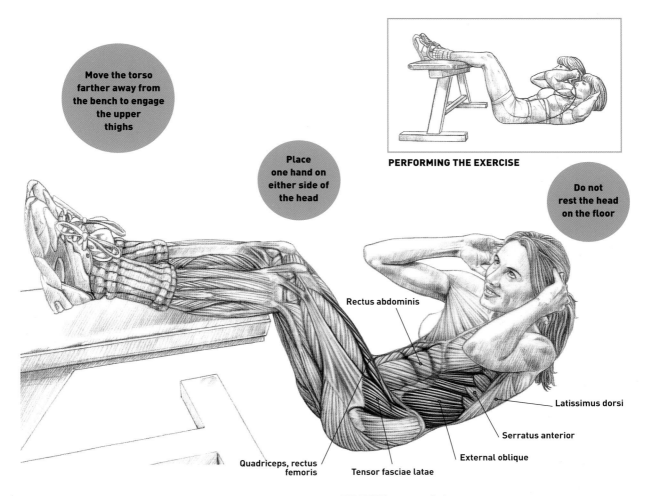

Rectus abdominis

Latissimus dorsi

Serratus anterior

External oblique

Tensor fasciae latae

Quadriceps, rectus femoris

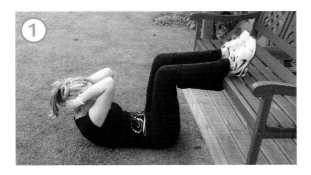

VARIATION: arms out in front

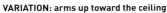

VARIATION: arms up toward the ceiling

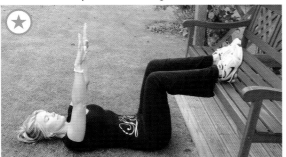

VARIATION: performing the exercise with arms toward ceiling

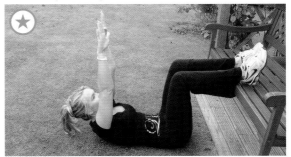

Oblique Crunch, Feet on the Floor or a Bench

Targets   Works the rectus abdominis and especially the external and internal obliques. This helps chisel the torso near the ribs to make the waist slimmer.

Repetitions   Do 3 or 4 sets of 20 to 30 repetitions.

Your coach's advice   Do not let your belly push out. When you inhale, just as when you exhale, engage your abdominal muscles and pull your navel in toward your spine.

Breathing   Exhale as you raise your torso and inhale as you lower it.

Warning   Be careful to keep your lower back firmly pressed into the floor. Keep your head in line with your spine. When your torso is lifted up, the upper part of your body should form a C shape.

Key to the exercise   Holding your arms in front of you and bringing them to the outside of your knees will make the exercise easier for the obliques. This exercise requires a small range of motion. For more advanced work, you can keep your hands behind your head, with one leg lifted and the foot of the other leg resting on the floor or on a bench. This way, the elbow initiates the movement toward the knee of the lifted leg. This movement works the obliques harder since you have to roll up more.

1. Lie on your back with bent legs and feet flat on the floor or on a bench. Hold your arms straight out in front and to one side of your body or by your ears.

2. As you exhale, contract your abdominal muscles and lift your head off the floor while lifting your upper back. Keep your lower back pressed into the floor. Touch the side of your knees with your hands.

3. As you inhale, return to the starting position, but do not rest your head on the floor. Repeat on the other side, alternating sides until you have completed your set.

Variation   To accentuate the work of the obliques, try to touch one knee with the opposite elbow. With your legs on the floor or on a bench, cross one ankle over the knee of the opposite leg. Roll up and bring the opposite elbow toward the knee of the crossed leg. Pay attention to the position of your hands behind your head: The fingers should not be interlaced and should not pull on your neck. If you choose this variation, then do not alternate sides. Instead, do a complete set on one side, and then switch legs so you can do a set on the other side.

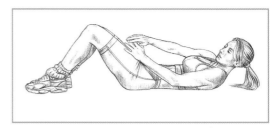

STARTING POSITION

Contract the abdominal wall throughout the exercise

Do not rest the head on the floor

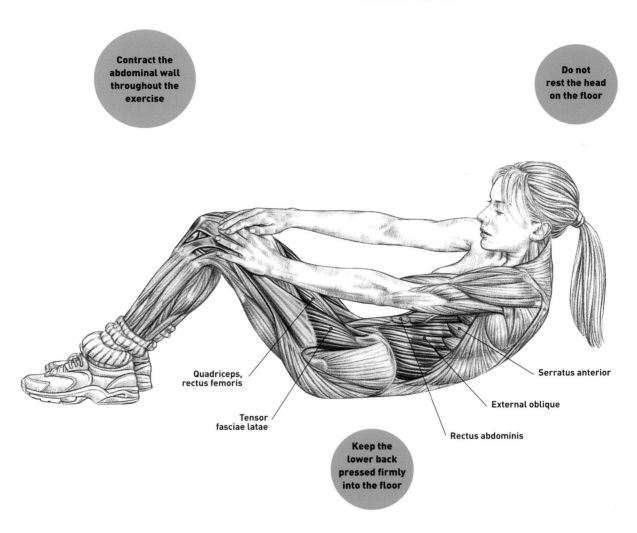

Quadriceps, rectus femoris

Serratus anterior

External oblique

Tensor fasciae latae

Rectus abdominis

Keep the lower back pressed firmly into the floor

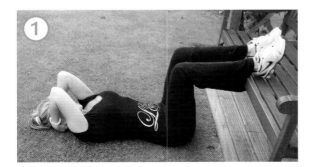

①

VARIATION: feet on a bench, elbow toward the opposite knee

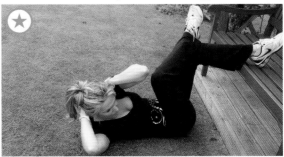

★

Oblique Crunch, Legs Raised

Targets   Works the rectus abdominis and especially the internal and external obliques. This helps chisel the torso near the ribs to make the waist slimmer.

Repetitions   Do 3 or 4 sets of 20 to 30 repetitions.

Your coach's advice   Tighten your abdominal wall like a corset and pay attention to your breathing: Exhale fully and regularly during the upward movement and inhale just as deeply and regularly during the downward movement.

Breathing   Exhale as you raise your torso and inhale as you lower it. You should not hold your breath and you should not take short, rapid breaths.

Warning   Do not pull on your cervical spine (be aware of the position of your hands), and do not make abrupt movements (the contraction of the abdominal muscles is what helps you roll up your spine and lift your torso gradually).

Key to the exercise   Lifting your legs up and having your thighs in a vertical position will help you keep your lumbar spine pressed into the floor. You may cross your ankles for greater stability in your legs. The farther apart you hold your elbows, the more this exercise will recruit your obliques.

1. Lie with your back pressed into the floor and your hands behind your head. Lift your legs so that your thighs are in a vertical position and bend your knees at 90 degrees. Cross your ankles.

2. As you exhale, contract your abdominal muscles and lift your upper torso by pulling your head and shoulders off the floor. Bring one elbow toward the opposite knee. (Ideally, the elbow should come slightly to the outside of the knee to work your waist and obliques most effectively. But depending on your ability level, you can bring the elbow close to or a little farther from the knee.)

3. As you inhale, lower to the starting position but do not rest your head on the floor. Repeat the exercise on the other side and continue alternating until you finish the set.

Variation   You can keep one leg bent with the foot on the floor or on a bench, and rest the ankle of the opposite leg on the thigh (see pages 60-61). As you exhale, roll up your spine and bring the opposite elbow toward the knee of the lifted leg. Do an entire set on this side and then switch to the other side instead of alternating throughout the set.

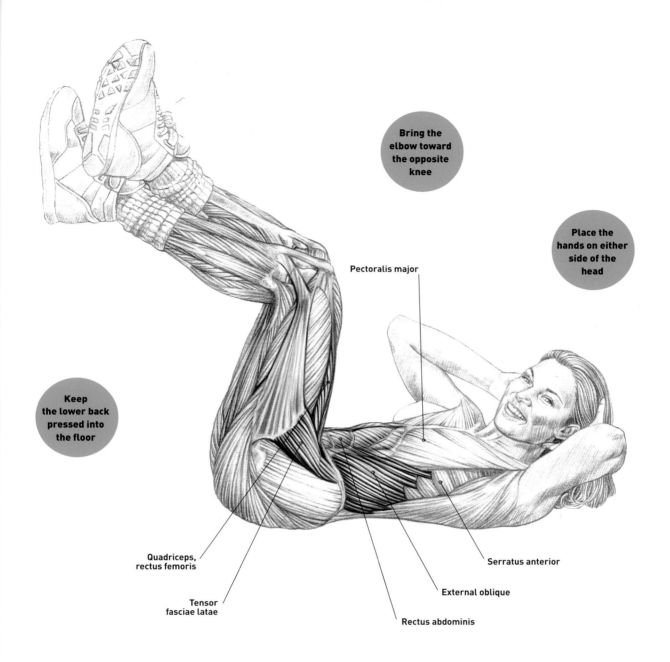

Bring the elbow toward the opposite knee

Place the hands on either side of the head

Keep the lower back pressed into the floor

Pectoralis major

Quadriceps, rectus femoris

Tensor fasciae latae

Rectus abdominis

External oblique

Serratus anterior

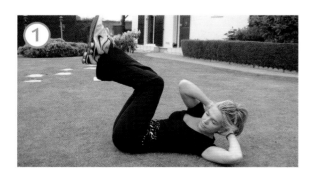

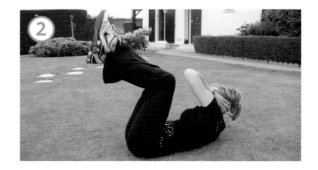

Leg Extension

Targets   Works the rectus abdominis (upper abdominal muscle), the obliques (external and internal), and the upper thigh muscles (tensor fasciae latae and rectus femoris).

Repetitions   Do 3 or 4 sets of 20 to 30 repetitions.

Your coach's advice   Your elbows should not be too close together (you could end up arching your back and injuring your lumbar spine) or too far apart (your back could collapse, bringing your shoulders close to your ears, and thus injuring your neck). Ideally, you should be able to round your back slightly throughout the exercise while keeping your shoulders well away from your ears.

Breathing   Exhale as you straighten your legs and inhale as you bend them.

Warning   The lower your legs are, the harder the exercise will be. However, there is no point in holding the legs too low since you also want to avoid engaging your lumbar spine.

Key to the exercise   Contract your abdominal muscles tightly to protect your lumbar spine, and concentrate on your abdominal wall. At the end of a set, you should feel a burning sensation that tells you your muscles have really been working.

1   Lie back with your elbows directly below your shoulders and your forearms and palms resting on the floor. Your legs should be bent and your feet should be flat on the floor. Contract your abdominal muscles.

2   As you exhale, straighten your legs with pointed or flexed feet (flexing your feet will engage the thigh muscles more).

3   As you inhale, return to the starting position without resting your feet on the floor. Do 20 to 30 repetitions slowly with no abrupt movements. Be sure to breathe deeply throughout the exercise.

Variation   To make this exercise more intense, keep your legs straight for 12 seconds while you squeeze your abdominal wall as hard as you can. Do not hold your breath, and bend your legs again as you inhale.

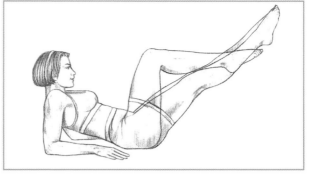

Keep the shoulders away from the ears

PERFORMING THE EXERCISE

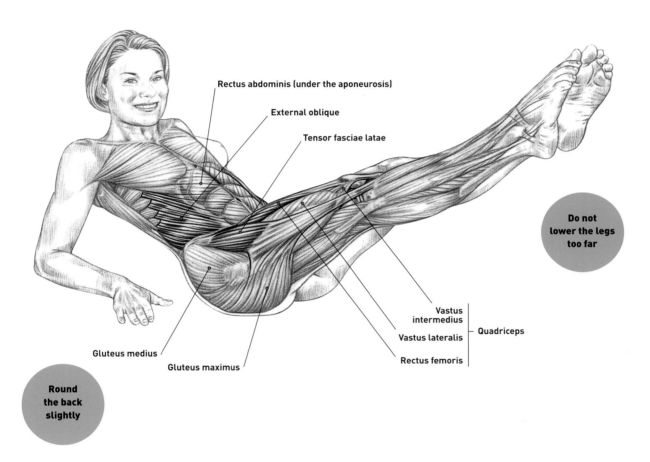

Rectus abdominis (under the aponeurosis)

External oblique

Tensor fasciae latae

Do not lower the legs too far

Vastus intermedius

Vastus lateralis — Quadriceps

Rectus femoris

Gluteus medius

Gluteus maximus

Round the back slightly

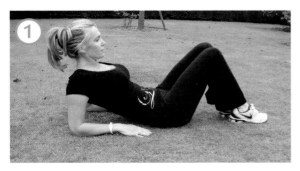

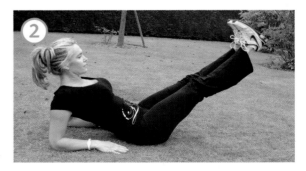

Reverse Crunch

Targets   Works the rectus abdominis as well as the internal and external oblique muscles.

Repetitions   Do 3 sets of 20 repetitions.

Your coach's advice   When done regularly (at least twice each week), sets of 12 to 20 repetitions provide great results if the exercise is done slowly while controlling the movement and concentrating on engaging the abdominal wall. The exercise should not be jerky; it should be fluid, especially during the descent.

Breathing   Exhale as you lift the legs and pelvis, and inhale as you lower them.

Warning   Do not lift up too high (this is not the candlestick exercise)! If you have trouble controlling your descent, which should be slow and gradual, then do not raise your pelvis as high, or do a variation with a smaller range of motion (bent knees).

Key to the exercise   What makes this exercise so effective is the control required and the engagement of the abdominal wall. When you raise and lower your legs, your abdomen should be tight and you should pull your navel in toward your spine.

1. Lie on your back with your legs up toward the ceiling and your arms alongside your body. Your palms should be touching the floor.

2. Contract your abdominal muscles tightly and then exhale as you gradually lift your buttocks and raise your pelvis and legs up in the air.

3. Relax slowly as you inhale. As soon as the pelvis touches the floor, repeat the exercise. Continue until you have completed your set.

Variation   In this exercise, your legs are basically straight, depending on the flexibility in your hamstring muscles (backs of the thighs). If you have difficulty straightening your legs or controlling your descent, then bend your legs, squeeze your knees together, and place your heels close to your buttocks. The range of motion will be smaller this way (the back remains pressed into the floor), and you will engage your lower abdominal muscles more. If this exercise is difficult for you, then try placing your hands underneath your buttocks. This will keep you from engaging your lumbar muscles unnecessarily.

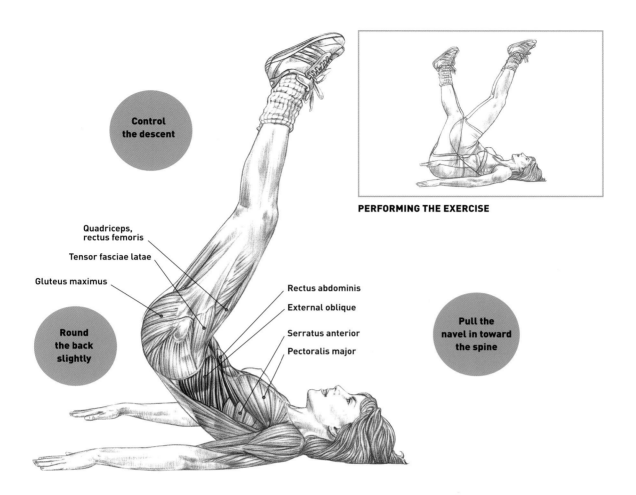

Control the descent

PERFORMING THE EXERCISE

Quadriceps, rectus femoris

Tensor fasciae latae

Gluteus maximus

Rectus abdominis

External oblique

Serratus anterior

Pectoralis major

Round the back slightly

Pull the navel in toward the spine

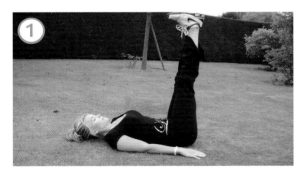

1

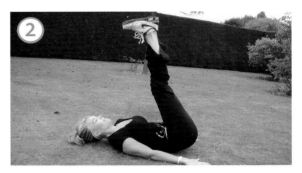

2

VARIATION: with bent legs

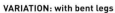
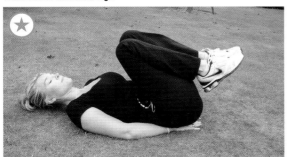

VARIATION: performing the exercise with bent legs

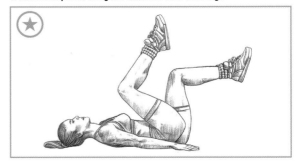

Bicycle

Targets   Works the rectus abdominis (upper abdominal muscle) and the internal and external oblique muscles, as well as the upper thigh muscles (tensor fasciae latae and rectus femoris).

Repetitions   Do 3 or 4 sets of 20 to 30 repetitions.

Your coach's advice   Always do this exercise slowly with no abrupt movements. It is better to do fewer repetitions while taking your time than to rush through it. Even though the exercise is more intense when the legs are closer to the floor, it is better to keep your legs higher than to compensate with your lumbar spine.

Breathing   You can inhale and exhale over one complete bicycle movement (one leg straightens and then the other), or you can exhale as you straighten one leg and inhale as you straighten the other leg.

Warning   At the first sign of discomfort in your lower back, check your position: Your torso should be straight, your back should be slightly rounded, and your pelvis should be tilted back (see page 30).

Key to the exercise   Begin the exercise with your legs as close to the floor as possible without arching your back. Then when the burning becomes too intense or you feel you are starting to compensate with your lower back, lift your legs a little higher so you can finish the set.

1. Lie back with your elbows directly underneath your shoulders and your forearms and palms resting on the floor. Bend your legs, pick your feet up off the floor, and contract your abdominal muscles.

2. As you exhale, straighten one leg with the foot flexed or pointed (keeping the foot flexed will work the thigh muscles more). Then, as you inhale, bend that leg as you straighten the other leg.

3. Continue alternating in this bicycling motion until you finish the set.

Variation   To make this exercise more intense, you can make a small up-and-down striking motion with your straight leg before you bend it and bring it back in. You can also do a true pedaling motion by moving the leg from high to low at the same time that you straighten then bend it. You can also pedal backward (from low to high).

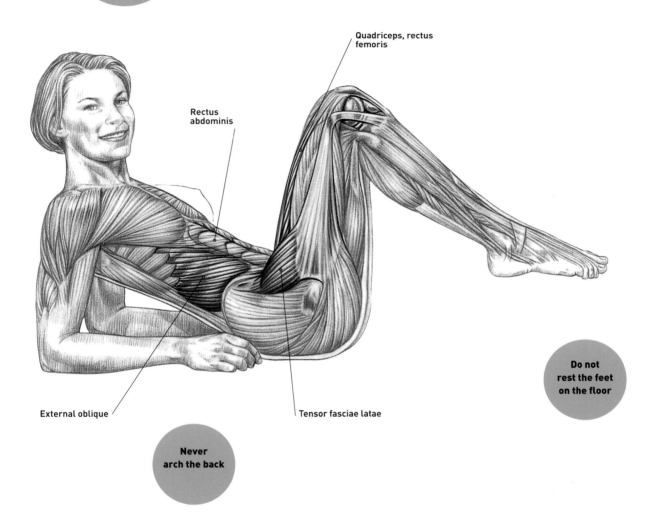

Keep the shoulders down and away from the ears

Quadriceps, rectus femoris

Rectus abdominis

External oblique

Tensor fasciae latae

Do not rest the feet on the floor

Never arch the back

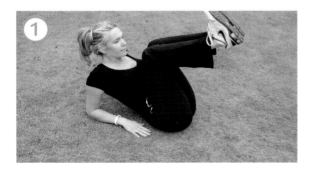

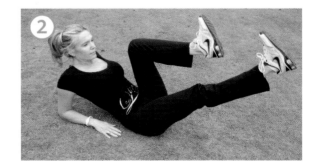

Oblique Bicycle

⊚ **Targets**   Works the rectus abdominis (upper abdominal muscle) and especially the oblique muscles (internal and external). It also works the upper thigh muscles (tensor fasciae latae and rectus femoris).

🕒 **Repetitions**   Do 3 or 4 sets of 20 to 30 repetitions.

👓 **Your coach's advice**   To perform this exercise correctly, roll up your spine by bringing your shoulders up off the floor each time your elbow approaches your knee. Pull in your navel toward your spine.

😮 **Breathing**   You can inhale and exhale over one complete bicycle movement (one elbow goes toward the opposite knee and then the other elbow goes toward the other knee), or you can exhale as you bring one elbow toward the opposite knee and inhale as you bring the other elbow to the other knee.

❗ **Warning**   Contract your abdominal muscles tightly to avoid engaging your lumbar region. Your shoulders should be off the floor, but your lower back and pelvis should stay as still as possible.

🔑 **Key to the exercise**   The closer you bring your elbow to the opposite knee, the better you will contract your oblique muscles and your rectus abdominis. Keep your elbows far apart from one another.

①   Lie on the floor with your hands on your ears or behind your neck (but without pulling on your cervical spine). Contract your abdominal muscles and lift your head and shoulders. Both legs are straight and off the floor with your feet flexed or pointed.

②   As you exhale, simultaneously bend one leg and bring the opposite elbow toward the knee. The torso pivots to the side and the elbows stay well apart toward the outside. As you inhale, straighten that leg, bend your other leg, and pivot your torso toward the other side, bringing the opposite elbow toward the bent knee.

③   Alternate in this pedaling motion until you finish the set.

⭐ **Variation**   To make this exercise more intense, you can make a small up-and-down striking motion with your straight leg before you bend it and bring it back in. You can also do this exercise with your arms out in front of you. Touch the outside of the foot of the bent leg with the hand on the same side or, to make it even harder, touch the inside of the foot of the bent leg with the hand of the opposite arm.

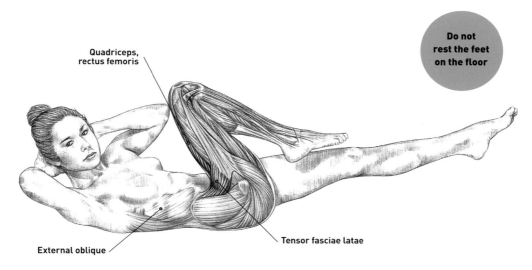

Quadriceps,
rectus femoris

**Do not
rest the feet
on the floor**

External oblique

Tensor fasciae latae

**Do not
interlace
the fingers as
shown here**

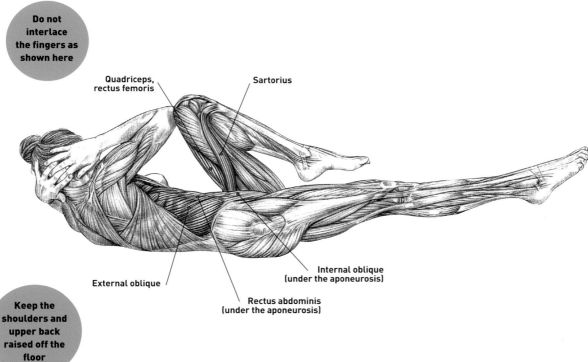

Quadriceps,
rectus femoris

Sartorius

External oblique

Rectus abdominis
(under the aponeurosis)

Internal oblique
(under the aponeurosis)

**Keep the
shoulders and
upper back
raised off the
floor**

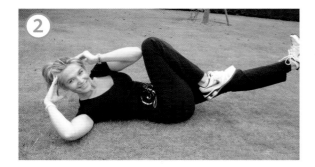

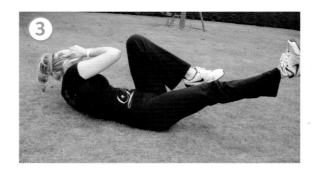

71

Sphinx

○ **Targets**   Stretches the abdominal wall and the lumbar region.

○ **Repetitions**   Hold the position for 30 to 60 seconds after each set of abdominal exercises.

○ **Your coach's advice**   This exercise stretches the entire abdominal wall. It is ideal for stretching the muscles after performing abdominal exercises. Focus on contracting your buttocks so that you do not compensate with your lumbar muscles. Keep your breathing slow and steady.

○ **Breathing**   Inhale and exhale deeply and calmly throughout the stretch.

○ **Warning**   You should not arch your back too much if you have lower back problems. Also, be sure to keep your shoulders down and away from your ears so that you do not tighten your neck muscles.

○ **Key to the exercise**   Keep your gaze focused upward (without cramping your neck) so that you can stretch your entire spine as well.

1 Lie on your front with straight legs and feet pointed backward. Bend your arms, and place your palms flat on the floor in front of your chest.

2 Push with your arms until they are straight and your torso is raised off the floor. Keep your head in line with your spine and contract your buttocks muscles.

3 Hold this position and take the time to breathe deeply during the stretch. Pay attention to the sensations in your body so that you do not engage your lumbar region.

★ **Variation**   If you feel that you arch your back too much when your arms are straight, then you can do this exercise with slightly bent arms. But if the stretch seems too easy, bring your hands closer to your hips by sliding your legs along the floor.

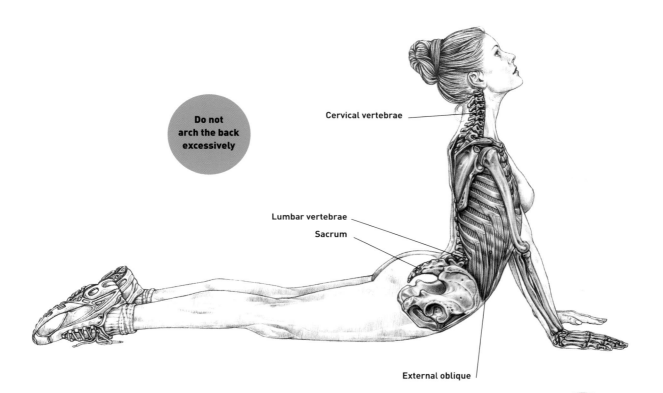

Do not bring the head too far backward

Do not arch the back excessively

Cervical vertebrae

Lumbar vertebrae

Sacrum

External oblique

Push with the palms of the hands

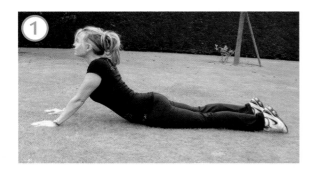

1

VARIATION: hands closer to hips

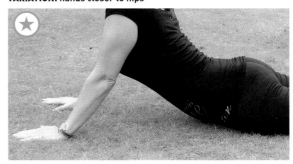

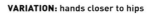

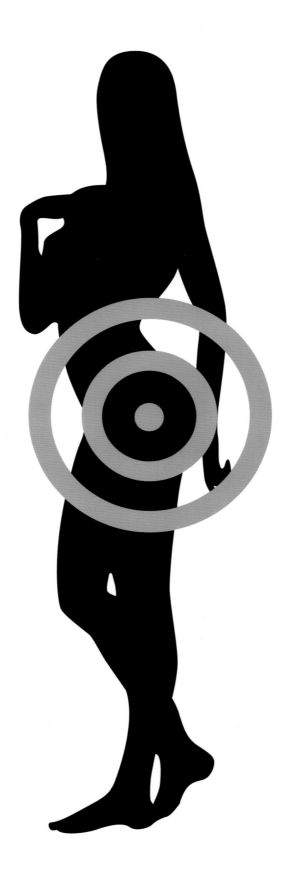

GOAL 3
Sculpt Your Butt

Leg Lift to the Side

Targets   Works the gluteus medius and is very effective at eliminating saddlebags.

Repetitions   Do 2 or 3 sets of 20 to 30 repetitions on each leg.

Your coach's advice   When done regularly (2 or 3 times each week) for 3 to 4 months, this exercise will help you get rid of excess fat on the side of your thighs, commonly called saddlebags. Once you have achieved noticeable results, maintain those results by continuing to do this exercise 1 or 2 times each week.

Breathing   Exhale as you raise your leg and inhale as you lower it.

Warning   Contract your abdominal muscles tightly to keep your balance and avoid arching your back, which could hurt your lumbar spine.

Key to the exercise   Keep the foot of the raised leg parallel to the floor to focus the work on the saddlebag area. Do not raise your leg too high, because then you will no longer be using the gluteus medius.

1. Lie on one side with your legs straight and stacked on top of one another. Place one elbow on the floor and use your other arm as support. Focus on contracting your buttocks and abdominal muscles tightly.

2. Raise your upper leg, keeping the foot parallel to the floor, and do 20 to 30 repetitions. Exhale as you raise your leg and inhale as you lower it.

3. Switch legs.

Variation   To make this exercise more intense, hold your leg in the raised position for about 5 seconds and continue exhaling. Then lower your leg. You can also use an ankle weight or resistance band. Finally, be aware that your leg position determines how much you work the front or the back part of the buttocks.

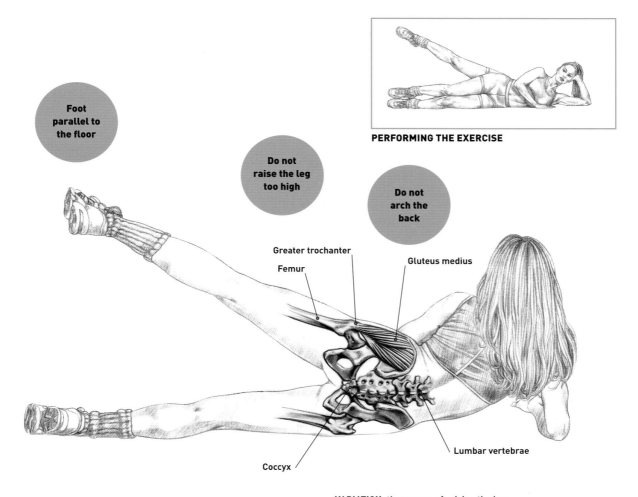

Foot parallel to the floor

Do not raise the leg too high

Do not arch the back

PERFORMING THE EXERCISE

Greater trochanter

Femur

Gluteus medius

Coccyx

Lumbar vertebrae

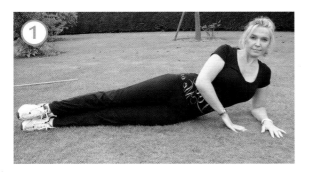

1

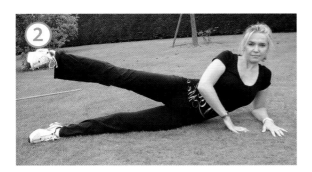

2

VARIATION: three ways of raising the leg

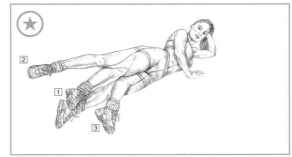

1. **Leg raised vertically**
2. **Leg raised slightly to the back**
3. **Leg raised slightly to the front**

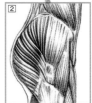
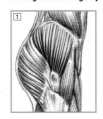
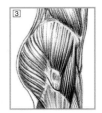

Leg Lift on the Belly

Targets   Works the gluteus maximus and the erector spinae muscles so you can have shapely buttocks and a beautiful lower back.

Repetitions   Do 2 or 3 sets of 20 to 30 repetitions on each leg.

Your coach's advice   This exercise is easy to do while you are doing something else, such as lying outdoors while flipping through a magazine. So try to do a few repetitions every chance you get, because the frequency of your workouts will determine your ultimate results!

Breathing   Exhale as you raise your leg and inhale as you lower it.

Warning   Contract your abdominal muscles very slightly and arch your back a little (but not too much). Your shoulders should be directly above your elbows and well away from your ears. Stretch your spine.

Key to the exercise   Point the foot of your raised leg to focus the work on the gluteus maximus or flex your foot to work your quadriceps more. Do not rest your leg on the floor between repetitions. Your foot should rest on the floor only at the end of a set.

1   Lie on your front, supporting yourself on your forearms. Arch your back slightly and gently lift one leg with the foot pointed.

2   As you exhale, raise your leg as high as you can without pinching your back. As you inhale, lower your leg without touching the floor and begin again until you have completed 20 to 30 repetitions.

3   Switch legs.

Variation   To make this exercise more intense, hold the leg in the raised position for 2 or 3 seconds as you exhale. Then lower the leg. You can also use ankle weights or a resistance band. Finally, you can bend your knee if you want to work the hamstrings (backs of the thighs) more.

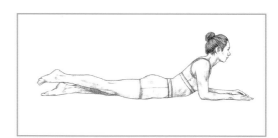

Foot pointed

Head in line with the spine

Erector spinae
(under the thoracolumbar fascia)

Long head

Biceps femoris

Short head

Semitendinosus

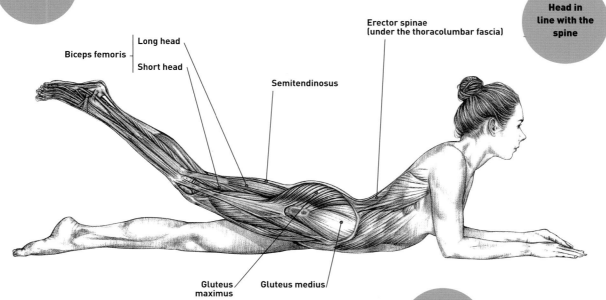

Gluteus maximus

Gluteus medius

Shoulders directly above the elbows

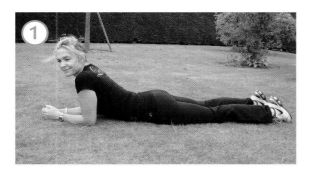

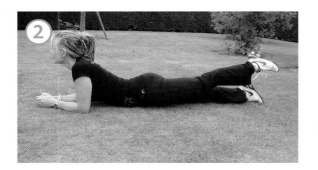

VARIATION: with bent knee

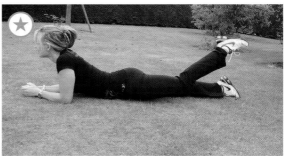

79

Leg Lift on the Knees

Targets   Works the gluteus maximus (curve of the buttocks).

Repetitions   Do 3 or 4 sets of 20 to 30 repetitions on each leg.

Your coach's advice   This exercise is effective when your body is aligned correctly. There is no point in raising your leg too high (because you could end up arching your back), and you must be careful to keep your torso very straight (to do this, contract your abdominal muscles and push on your forearms).

Breathing   Exhale as you raise the leg and inhale as you lower it.

Warning   Contract your abdominal muscles throughout the exercise to maintain your balance. Keep your head in line with your spine.

Key to the exercise   Keep your foot flexed as you raise it to stretch your calf and avoid contracting your thigh muscles.

1. On your knees with your elbows and forearms on the floor., your head should be in line with your body and your abdominal and buttocks muscles should be firmly contracted. Bring one knee forward to your chest.

2. As you exhale, raise your leg and straighten it behind you with the foot flexed or neutral. As you inhale, return to the starting position and bring the knee close to the chest. The leg does not touch the floor. Do 20 to 30 repetitions in this way.

3. Switch legs.

Variation   To make this exercise more intense, hold the leg in the raised position for 2 or 3 seconds as you exhale, and then lower the leg. You can also use a weight. If you want to work the inner thigh muscles and the gluteus medius (outside of the butt) more, keep your leg straight as you lower it toward the outside of the supporting leg instead of pulling it under your chest. This variation is excellent for recruiting muscles that are not used very often, so it will help you to avoid having your inner thighs touch each other.

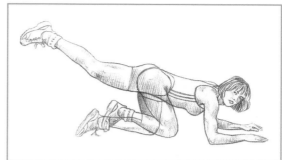

PERFORMING THE EXERCISE

Foot is flexed or neutral

Head in line with the spine

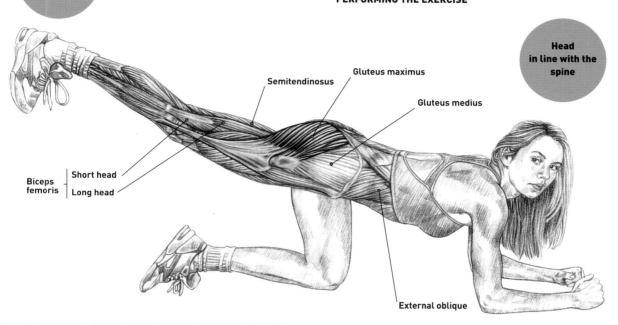

Semitendinosus

Gluteus maximus

Gluteus medius

Biceps femoris — Short head / Long head

External oblique

Shoulders directly above the elbows

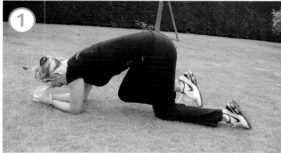

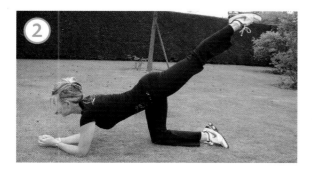

VARIATION: lowering the straight leg to the outside of the supporting leg

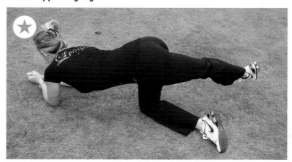

81

Leg Lift With a Bent Knee

Targets   Works the gluteus medius and the gluteus maximus (for a firm, rounded butt).

Repetitions   Do 3 or 4 sets of 20 to 30 repetitions on each leg.

Your coach's advice   Contract your buttocks tightly during the exercise. Even though this exercise already works the buttocks, consciously engaging them will help you recruit them even more.

Breathing   Exhale as you raise your leg and inhale as you lower it.

Warning   Tighten your abdominal muscles throughout the exercise to maintain your balance and avoid arching your back. Keep your head in line with your spine. Lower your leg with control. Do not raise your leg too high and do not lower it too quickly.

Key to the exercise   To engage the backs of the thighs (hamstrings) at the same time, just bend the working leg to 90 degrees. Bending it any more than that reduces the range of motion and could cause you to arch your back.

(1) Get on your knees and place your elbows and forearms on the floor. Keep your head in line with your body, and tighten your abdominal and buttocks muscles. Lift one leg off the floor.

(2) Exhale and lift the bent leg to 90 degrees behind you, keeping the foot flexed or neutral. Inhale and return to the starting position, but do not let your knee touch the floor. Do 20 to 30 repetitions in this way.

(3) Switch legs.

(★) **Variation**   To make this exercise more intense, hold your leg in the raised position for 2 or 3 seconds as you exhale, and then lower it. You can also use a weight. To engage your hamstrings (backs of the thighs) more, start the exercise with a straight leg. Now bend the leg and raise it up. Then straighten the leg and lower it.

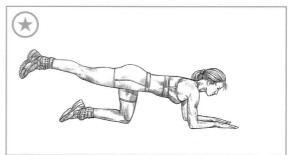

PERFORMING THE EXERCISE

The hip is above the knee

The head is in line with the spine

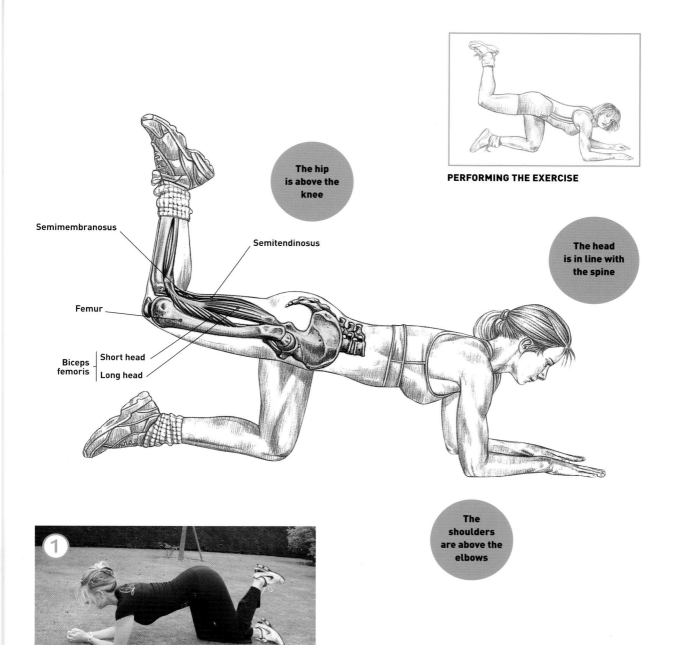

Semimembranosus

Semitendinosus

Femur

Biceps femoris — Short head

Long head

The shoulders are above the elbows

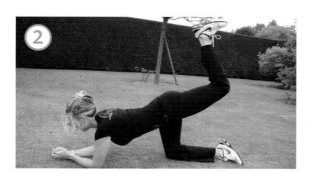

1

2

VARIATION: starting with a straight leg

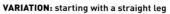

Opposite Arm and Leg Raise

Targets   Improves your balance and increases strength, especially in the gluteus maximus (rounded, posterior part of the butt) and all the muscles of the lower back (quadratus lumborum and erector spinae muscles).

Repetitions   Hold the position for 30 to 40 seconds, 3 or 4 times on each side.

Your coach's advice   Stabilization exercises are ideal for recruiting a large number of muscles and improving stability. However, it is critical that you pay attention to your posture since this is a static position. Be sure that your spine is lengthened perfectly.

Breathing   Inhale and exhale deeply and calmly throughout the exercise.

Warning   Tighten your abdominal muscles throughout the exercise to maintain your balance and avoid arching your back. Keep your head in line with your spine. Lengthening your straight leg and arm should help you maintain proper alignment.

Key to the exercise   Focus on contracting your buttocks and the muscles in your lower back. Lengthen your inhalations and exhalations as you hold the position.

1. Kneel on one leg and support yourself with the opposite arm. Inhale and slowly lift your other arm and leg in line with your body to form a straight line.

2. Hold the position while you inhale and exhale. Your abdominal wall should be slightly contracted and your head should be in line with your spine. Each time you exhale, stretch your leg backward and your arm forward a tiny bit.

3. Relax and switch sides.

Variation   You can do small up-and-down movements with your straight arm and leg while you hold the position. Be careful to control these movements and to use a small range of motion.

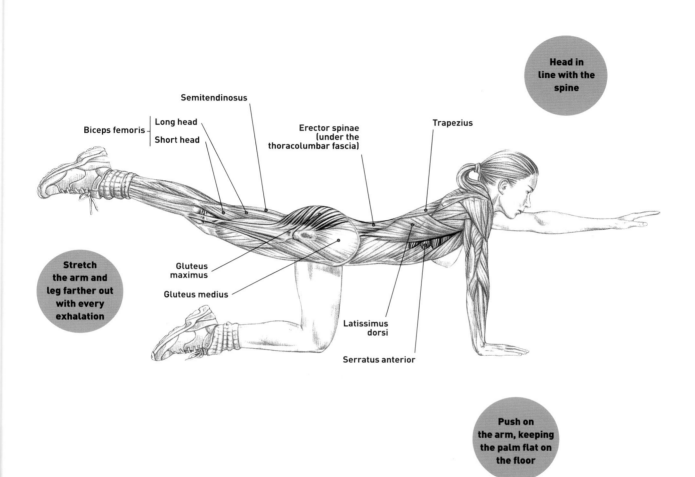

Semitendinosus

Biceps femoris — Long head
Short head

Erector spinae
(under the
thoracolumbar fascia)

Trapezius

Head in
line with the
spine

Stretch
the arm and
leg farther out
with every
exhalation

Gluteus
maximus

Gluteus medius

Latissimus
dorsi

Serratus anterior

Push on
the arm, keeping
the palm flat on
the floor

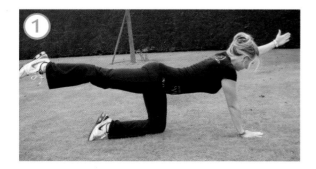

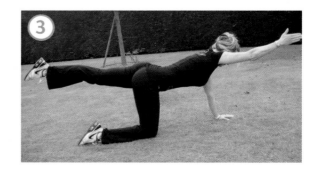

Side Leg Raise on the Knees

Targets   Works the gluteus medius and the gluteus minimus (which is located under the gluteus medius). Very effective at sculpting the outside of the thigh to eliminate saddlebags.

Repetitions   Do 3 or 4 sets of 20 to 30 repetitions on each leg.

Your coach's advice   Be careful not to twist your spine. Your arms should be straight and you should push equally on both hands, keeping your head in line with your spine. Tighten your abdominal muscles for greater stability.

Breathing   Exhale as you raise the leg and inhale as you lower it.

Warning   Hip abduction is physiologically limited, so there is no point in forcing things to try to lift your thigh above horizontal. It will not make the exercise any better!

Key to the exercise   If you are having trouble with your balance, put your hands a little bit farther than shoulder-width apart. Not only will this help your stability, but you will focus the work more on your buttocks.

1. Get on your hands and knees. Keep your arms straight, your palms flat on the floor, and your head in line with your body. Contract your abdominal and buttocks muscles tightly.

2. As you exhale, raise one knee to the side, keeping the leg bent. Your arms should be straight and your pelvis should not move. As you inhale, come back to the starting position, but do not rest your leg on the floor. Do 20 to 30 repetitions in this way.

3. Switch legs.

★ **Variation**   To make this exercise more intense, hold your leg in the raised position for 2 or 3 seconds as you exhale, and then lower it. You can also straighten your leg with your foot flexed and then bend it again to bring it back to the starting position. Your movements should be fluid, with no jerky motions. If, however, you find this exercise too difficult, you can also do it while lying on your side.

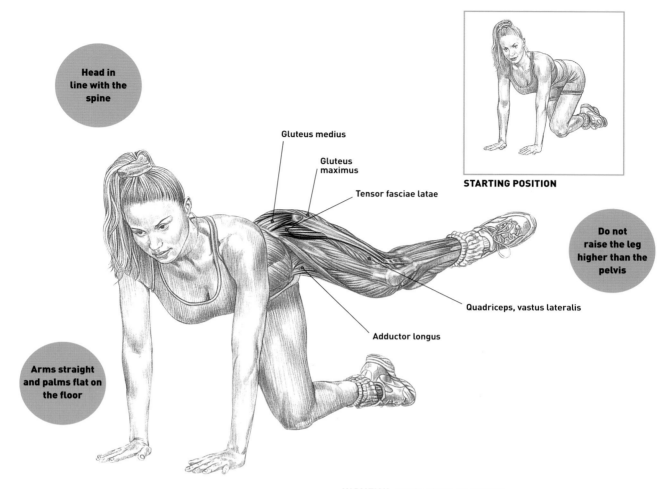

Head in line with the spine

Gluteus medius

Gluteus maximus

Tensor fasciae latae

STARTING POSITION

Do not raise the leg higher than the pelvis

Quadriceps, vastus lateralis

Adductor longus

Arms straight and palms flat on the floor

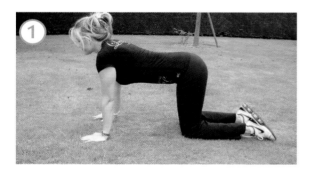

①

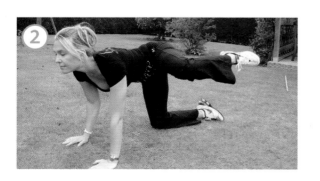

②

VARIATION: starting with a straight leg

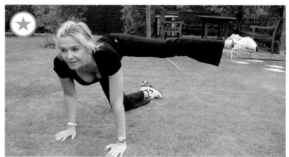

★

VARIATION: lying on the side

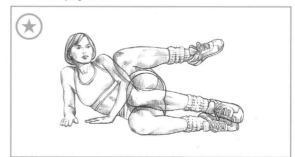

★

Bridge

Targets   Works the hamstrings and the lower part of the butt (gluteus maximus) to chisel the entire back of the leg.

Repetitions   Do 4 sets of 30 repetitions.

Your coach's advice   Throughout the exercise, keep looking at your chest so that you do not hurt your cervical spine.

Breathing   Exhale as you lift your pelvis up and inhale as you come down.

Warning   Do not raise your pelvis too high. Contract your buttocks and hamstring muscles firmly to avoid engaging your lumbar region.

Key to the exercise   Squeeze your knees together so you can better contract your hip adductors.

1   Lie on your back with your arms alongside your body and your palms flat on the floor. Keep your legs bent and the soles of your feet flat on the floor. Press your back firmly into the floor, inhale deeply, and bring your navel toward your spine.

2   Exhale as you lift your pelvis to form a straight line from your sternum to your knees. Press your shoulders into the floor and keep your knees pointing forward.

3   Inhale as you gently lower your torso with control. Then repeat the exercise without touching the floor.

Variation   To make the exercise more intense, you can hold the raised position for 12 seconds. However, you should not hold your breath. You can also do a series of up-and-down movements with a small range of motion (more dynamic than if you were lifting your torso all the way up).

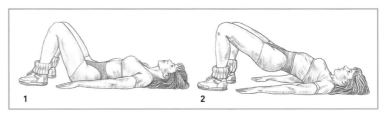

1. Starting position; 2. Performing the exercise

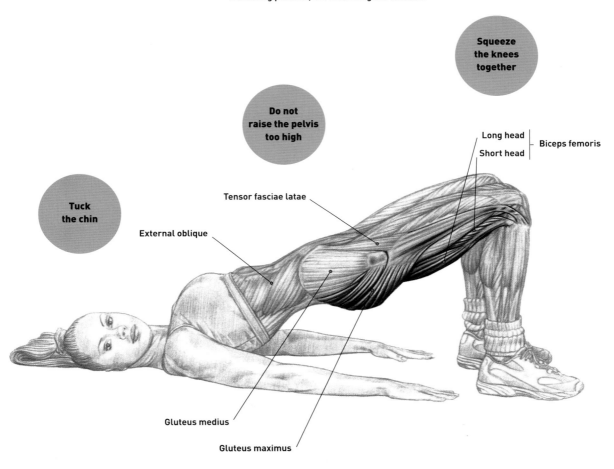

Squeeze the knees together

Do not raise the pelvis too high

Tuck the chin

Long head
Short head
Biceps femoris

Tensor fasciae latae

External oblique

Gluteus medius

Gluteus maximus

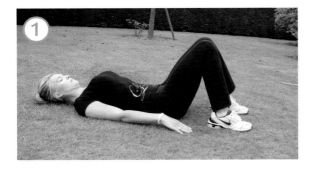

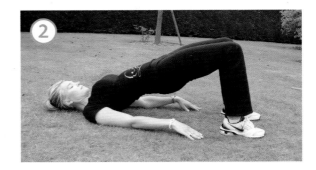

Bridge, Feet on a Bench

⊙ Targets   Intense hamstring work that also strengthens the gastrocnemius muscles (backs of the calves).

⏱ Repetitions   Do 4 sets of 30 repetitions.

👓 Your coach's advice   Tuck your chin and stretch out your upper back along the floor. Try to keep your shoulders as far apart from each other as possible and, in the raised position, open up your sternum.

😮 Breathing   Exhale as you raise your torso and inhale as you come down.

❗ Warning   To ensure that your body is at the proper distance from the bench, check that your legs are bent at a right angle in the starting position. Any closer and you risk arching your back excessively. Any farther away and you could lose your balance. Your knees, hips, and chest should be aligned in the raised position. Do not go any higher than that.

🔑 Key to the exercise   The exercise will be even more effective if you can support yourself using only your heels without pressing the soles of your feet into the bench, even in the raised position.

① Lie on the floor with your arms alongside your body and your palms on the floor. Keep your legs bent at a right angle and your feet resting on a bench. Your back should be pressed into the floor. Inhale deeply and bring your navel toward your spine.

② As you exhale, raise your pelvis to form a straight line from your sternum to your knees. Press your shoulders into the floor and keep your knees pointing forward.

③ Inhale as you gently lower your torso with control. Then, without touching the floor, repeat the exercise.

★ Variation   To increase the intensity of the exercise, you can hold the raised position for 4 or 5 seconds, but do not hold your breath. You can also do a series of up-and-down movements with a small range of motion (more dynamic than if you were lifting your torso all the way up). Or you can just squeeze your buttocks muscles rapidly while you are in the raised position.

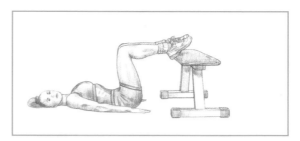

STARTING POSITION

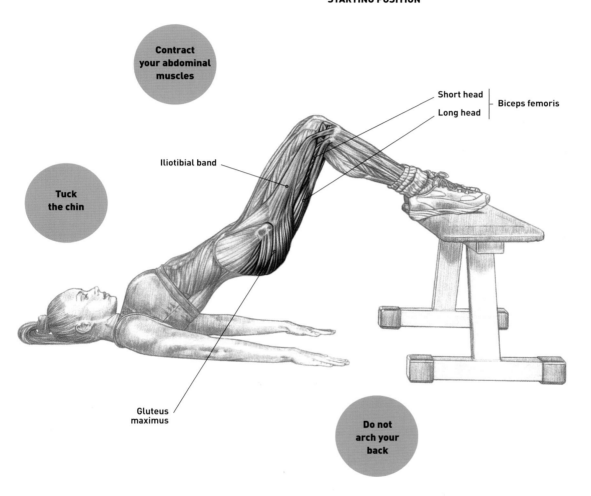

Contract your abdominal muscles

Tuck the chin

Iliotibial band

Short head
Long head
Biceps femoris

Gluteus maximus

Do not arch your back

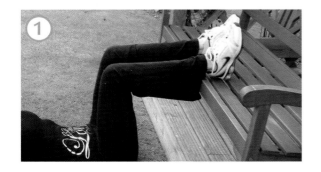

1

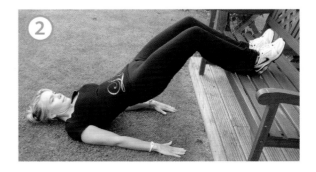

2

Bridge, One Leg Raised

Targets   Works the hamstrings and the lower buttocks (gluteus maximus) and is very effective at eliminating sagging.

Repetitions   Do 3 or 4 sets of 20 to 30 repetitions on each leg.

Your coach's advice   Push firmly on the supporting foot to help your balance. Tuck your chin and look at your chest. Your shoulders, arms, and palms also provide a stable base.

Breathing   Exhale as you raise your torso and inhale as you come down.

Warning   Do not raise your pelvis or your straight leg too high. Your hips should be aligned. Contract your buttocks and abdominal muscles to avoid engaging your lumbar region unnecessarily.

Key to the exercise   Keep the foot flexed to stretch the calf muscle of the straight leg.

1. Lie with your arms alongside your body and your palms on the floor. Press your back into the floor and keep one leg bent with the sole of the foot firmly pressed into the floor. The other leg is straight and held above the floor. Inhale deeply and bring your navel toward your spine.

2. As you exhale, raise your pelvis to form a straight line between your sternum, pelvis, knees, and the foot of the straight leg, as shown in the illustration. Press your shoulders into the floor and keep the knee of the supporting leg pointed forward. In the photo, the raised leg is lower, which is more difficult.

3. As you inhale, gently lower your torso with control. Repeat the movement without touching your torso to the floor. At the end of the set, switch legs.

Variation   To increase the intensity of the exercise, you can hold the raised position for 4 or 5 seconds, but do not hold your breath. Instead of doing a full set on one side and then the other, you can alternate doing bridges on the right and left legs during the same set. In this case, rest your back on the floor in between each repetition.

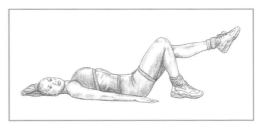

STARTING POSITION

Contract the abdominal muscles

Keep the pelvis aligned

Tuck the chin

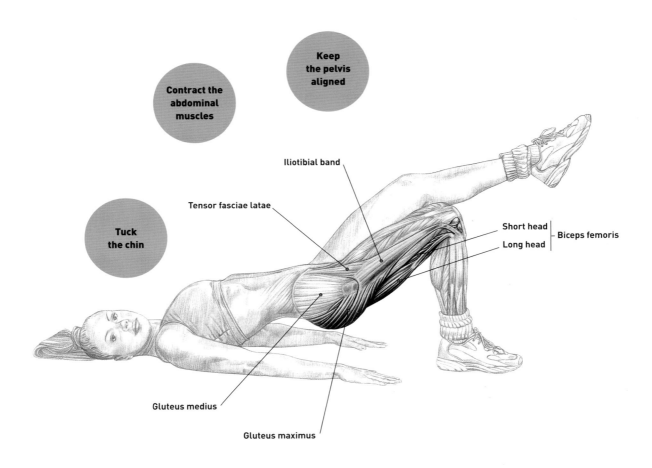

Iliotibial band

Tensor fasciae latae

Short head
Long head
Biceps femoris

Gluteus medius

Gluteus maximus

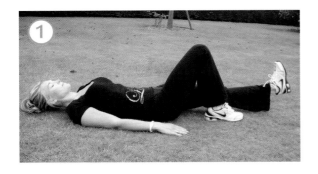

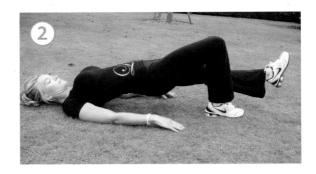

Lying Hamstring Stretch

Targets   When combined with strengthening exercises, this stretch helps define and elongate the back of the thigh.

Repetitions   Hold the stretch for 30 to 40 seconds. Do this stretch at the end of your buttocks and hamstring workouts.

Your coach's advice   If you are not flexible enough to straighten your legs, then you can bend the leg on the floor and the one in the air slightly, but you absolutely must not allow your butt to lift off the floor.

Breathing   Inhale and exhale deeply and calmly throughout the stretch.

Warning   Never force things when you stretch, and focus on your breathing throughout the stretch. You can pull gently on the leg to bring it gradually closer to you, but you should never make jerky movements.

Key to the exercise   To stretch the calves and hamstrings the most, flex the foot of the leg in the air.

1. Lie on your back with one leg straight and resting on the floor. Bend the other leg and bring it toward your abdomen. Place your hands on the back of the thigh of the bent leg.

2. Gently straighten that leg and try to lengthen it upward as much as you can.

3. Set that leg on the floor and switch legs.

Variation   Depending on your flexibility, you may need to bend the leg on the floor and the leg in the air a little bit. Stretching with a bent leg will recruit the gluteus maximus more, and stretching with a straight leg will recruit the hamstrings more.

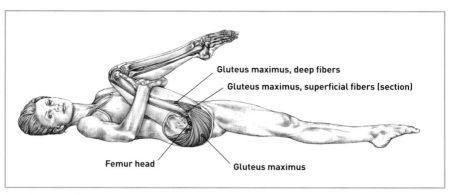

Gluteus maximus, deep fibers

Gluteus maximus, superficial fibers (section)

Femur head

Gluteus maximus

STARTING POSITION

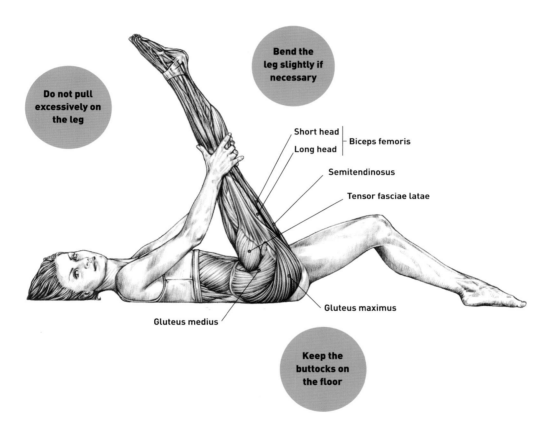

Do not pull excessively on the leg

Bend the leg slightly if necessary

Short head
Long head
— Biceps femoris

Semitendinosus

Tensor fasciae latae

Gluteus maximus

Gluteus medius

Keep the buttocks on the floor

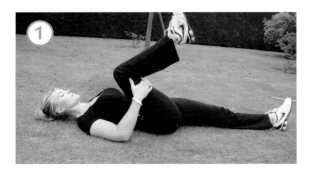

①

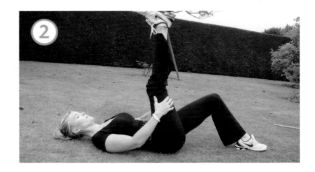

②

Buttocks Stretch

○ **Targets**   This intense stretch for the gluteus maximus also relaxes the lumbar region.

○ **Repetitions**   Hold the stretch for 30 to 40 seconds on each side. Do this stretch at the end of your buttocks and hamstrings workouts.

○ **Your coach's advice**   Stretches are too often thought of as just a way to prevent muscle aches, and they are quite often neglected. However, it has been proven that, when combined with strengthening exercises, they enhance the effectiveness of those exercises. You should always allow some time for stretching at the end of a workout.

○ **Breathing**   Inhale and exhale deeply and calmly throughout the stretch.

○ **Warning**   Spread your fingers wide apart on the floor for better support and to help you stretch your spinal column up to the ceiling. Pull in your navel to create more space between your torso and thigh to promote rotation.

○ **Key to the exercise**   Keep your back straight. This will help you not only to focus more on the gluteus maximus but also to better oxygenate your muscles.

1 Sit on the floor. Bend your right leg and put that foot on the outside of your straight left leg.

2 Put your right hand flat on the floor behind your buttocks. Press the back of your left arm against the outside of the bent knee. Your torso should be very straight; your spine should be lengthened toward the ceiling.

3 Hold the position to stretch your buttocks, remembering to breathe deeply. You can apply gentle pressure with your elbow to intensify the stretch on your leg. Switch legs.

★ Variation   To accentuate the stretch in the lumbar region (erector spinae) as well as in the oblique and neck muscles, you can rotate your torso even more, open up your shoulders and sternum, and turn your head toward the back, looking behind your shoulder.

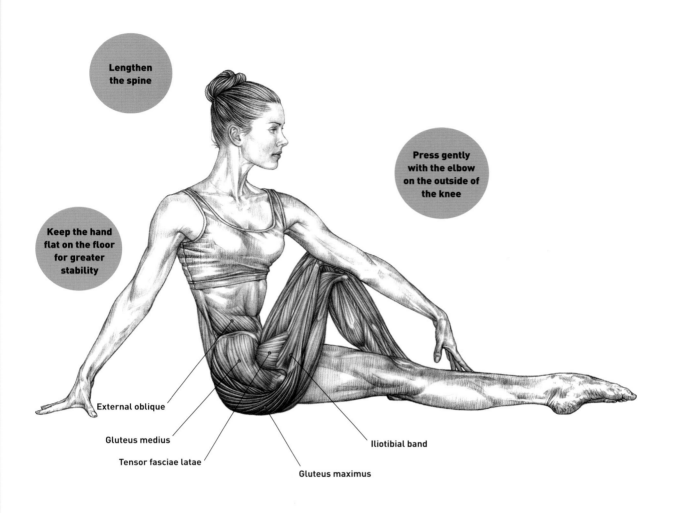

Lengthen the spine

Press gently with the elbow on the outside of the knee

Keep the hand flat on the floor for greater stability

External oblique

Gluteus medius

Tensor fasciae latae

Gluteus maximus

Iliotibial band

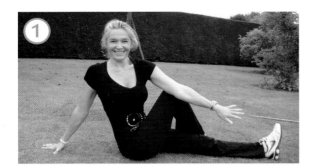

1

VARIATION: to accentuate the stretch in the lumbar region

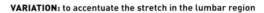

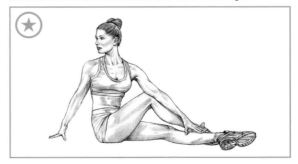

Leg Extension to the Back

Targets   Works the gluteus maximus (curved part of the butt).

Repetitions   Do 3 or 4 sets of 20 to 30 repetitions on each leg.

Your coach's advice   This exercise is also excellent for improving your balance. Crossing your arms in front of you will help stabilize your body, but in order to hold the position, you will have to recruit your abdominal wall.

Breathing   Exhale as you raise your leg and inhale as you lower it.

Warning   There is no point in raising your leg too high because that will cause you to arch your back. Your torso should remain straight.

Key to the exercise   The gluteus maximus works as you raise the leg and as you lower it, provided that you control the speed and the movement is slow and gradual.

1) Stand with straight legs and tilt your pelvis to the back (see page 30).

2) Support yourself on one leg with your foot flat on the floor. Contract your abdominal and buttocks muscles to maintain your balance. As you exhale, lift your other straight leg to the back and cross your arms in front of you (or you can start with your arms already crossed in front).

3) Inhale and return to the starting position, but do not set your foot on the floor. Repeat the exercise, and at the end of your set, switch legs.

Variation   To make this exercise more intense, you can use weights or a resistance band. If you are having balance problems, you can do this exercise with your hands on a wall or you can use a stick. If you are using a stick, you can bend your leg and lift it in front of you before you straighten it behind you. This way you can also work the quadriceps.

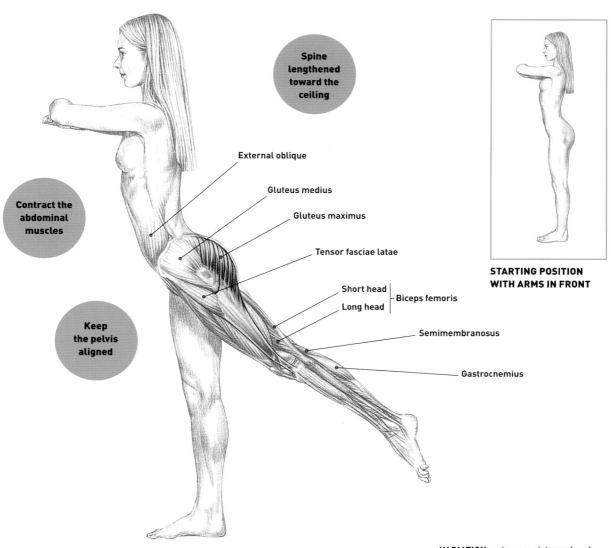

Spine lengthened toward the ceiling

Contract the abdominal muscles

Keep the pelvis aligned

External oblique

Gluteus medius

Gluteus maximus

Tensor fasciae latae

Short head — Biceps femoris
Long head

Semimembranosus

Gastrocnemius

STARTING POSITION WITH ARMS IN FRONT

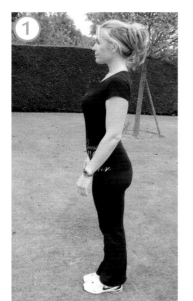

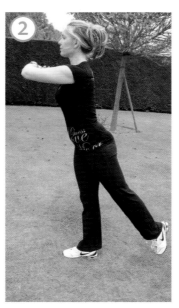

VARIATION: using a resistance band

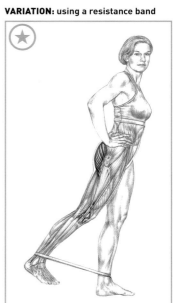

Leg Extension to the Side

Targets   This exercise tones and firms the gluteus medius as well as the gluteus minimus (which is located underneath the gluteus medius). It is particularly good for the saddlebag area.

Repetitions   Do 3 or 4 sets of 20 to 30 repetitions on each leg.

Your coach's advice   To keep your balance, and especially to keep your pelvis aligned, you must recruit your abdominal wall.

Breathing   Exhale as you raise your leg and inhale as you lower it.

Warning   It serves no purpose to lift your leg too high because this could cause you to move your hips. Keep your torso very straight.

Key to the exercise   For this exercise to be effective, you must keep your leg in line, pelvis straight, hips parallel, and foot flexed.

1. Stand with your legs together and place one hand on your waist and the other on a support (such as a wall) to provide stability. Gently lift one foot off the floor.

2. As you exhale, contract your buttocks and lift your straight leg to the side. Keep your foot flexed and parallel to the floor to focus the work on the outer part of the leg.

3. As you inhale, return to the starting position, but do not set your foot on the floor. Repeat the exercise. At the end of the set, switch legs.

★ **Variation**   You can also use a stick as a support (placed to the side or in front of you). To make this exercise more intense, you can use weights or a resistance band. If you do not have any balance problems and this exercise is easy for you, you can do it with your arms crossed in front of you. If you straighten your leg slightly in front, you will recruit the tensor fasciae latae more. If you straighten it slightly behind, you will recruit the upper part of the gluteus maximus more.

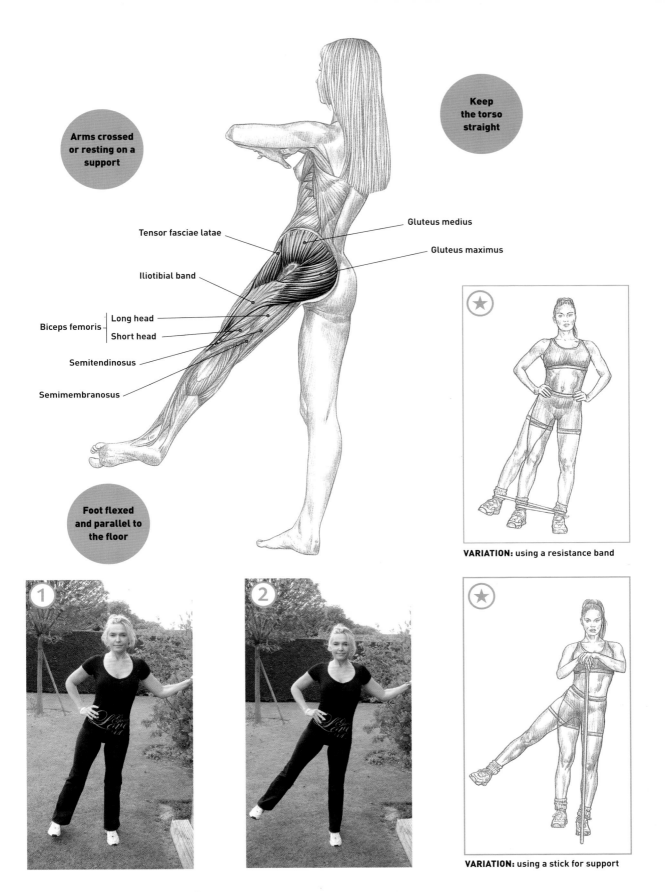

Arms crossed or resting on a support

Keep the torso straight

Tensor fasciae latae

Gluteus medius

Gluteus maximus

Iliotibial band

Biceps femoris — Long head

Short head

Semitendinosus

Semimembranosus

Foot flexed and parallel to the floor

VARIATION: using a resistance band

VARIATION: using a stick for support

Lateral Leg Curl

⊙ **Targets**   This exercise tones and firms the gluteus medius as well as the gluteus minimus (which is located underneath the gluteus medius). The final bending movement recruits the gluteus maximus. So this exercise works all the muscles in the buttocks.

🕐 **Repetitions**   Do 3 or 4 sets of 20 to 30 repetitions on each leg.

∞ **Your coach's advice**   Do not raise your leg too high; your pelvis should stay straight and still. Try to hold your body in the same position throughout the exercise. Only the lower part of the leg moves. To do this, you must remember to tighten your abdominal muscles.

☺ **Breathing**   Exhale as you bend your leg and inhale as you straighten it.

❗ **Warning**   Be careful not to move your hips. Keep your back straight, pelvis toward the front, and hips parallel throughout the exercise.

🔑 **Key to the exercise**   For this exercise to be effective, you must keep your leg in line, pelvis straight, hips parallel, and foot flexed.

① Stand with your legs together and place one hand on your waist and the other on a stick for support.

② As you exhale, contract your buttocks and lift one straight leg to the side with the foot flexed and parallel to the floor to focus the work on the outer part of the leg.

③ On the next exhalation, bend the lower part of the leg and bring the heel toward your buttocks, still keeping the foot flexed. As you inhale, straighten your leg and begin again. At the end of your set, switch legs.

⭐ **Variation**   Depending on how you feel and if you have no balance problems, you can do this exercise with your arms crossed in front of you or with your hands on your hips. See what works best for you. Putting your hands on your hips allows you to control the alignment of your pelvis during the exercise.

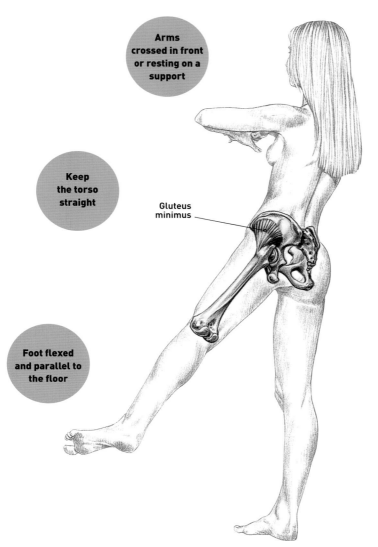

Arms crossed in front or resting on a support

Keep the torso straight

Gluteus minimus

Foot flexed and parallel to the floor

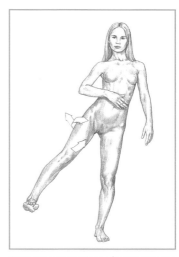

Abduction movements (extending the leg to the side) as well as flexing and internally rotating the leg work the gluteus minimus and the front part of the gluteus medius.

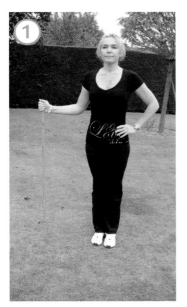

1

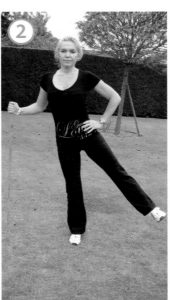

2

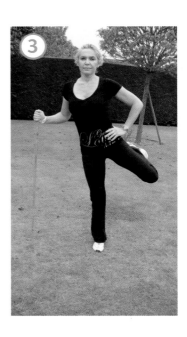

3

103

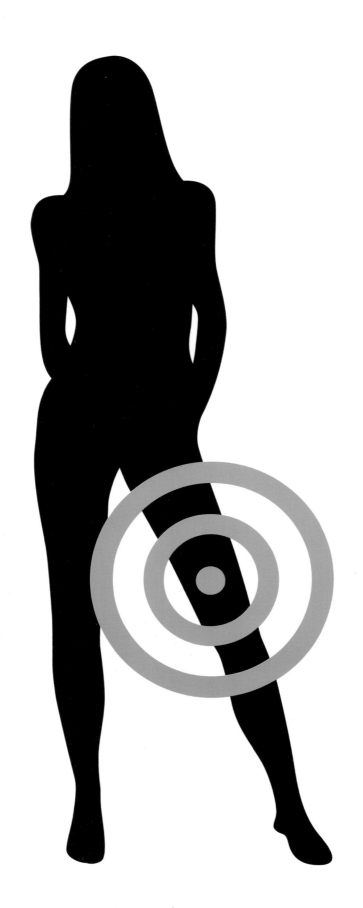

GOAL 4
Tone Your Legs

Standing Knee Raise

Targets   Works the quadriceps and the tensor fasciae latae; tones the front of the leg.

Repetitions   Do 3 or 4 sets of 20 to 30 repetitions on each leg.

Your coach's advice   To maintain your balance and keep your pelvis facing forward, engage your abdominal wall and contract your buttocks muscles.

Breathing   Exhale as you raise your leg, and inhale as you lower it.

Warning   Do not arch your back; before starting, tilt your pelvis backward (see page 30).

Key to the exercise   To make this exercise most effective, work dynamically as you lift your leg (that is, do it as fast as possible), but control how you lower your leg, and do it slowly.

1. Stand with your legs together, hands on your hips, and back very straight. Support yourself on one leg. Bend the other leg so that the ball of your foot is touching the floor.

2. Exhale, contract your buttocks, and lift your bent leg in front of you up to a right angle so that your thigh is parallel or a little past parallel to the floor.

3. Inhale as you return to the starting position, but do not set your foot on the floor. Begin again, and at the end of your set, switch legs.

⭐ **Variation**   You can also use a support during this exercise (one hand on a stick or a wall). To make this exercise more intense, you can use weights. At the end of the exercise, you can also hold the raised position for 2 or 3 seconds or bring your leg even closer to your chest. This will also stretch your buttocks muscles.

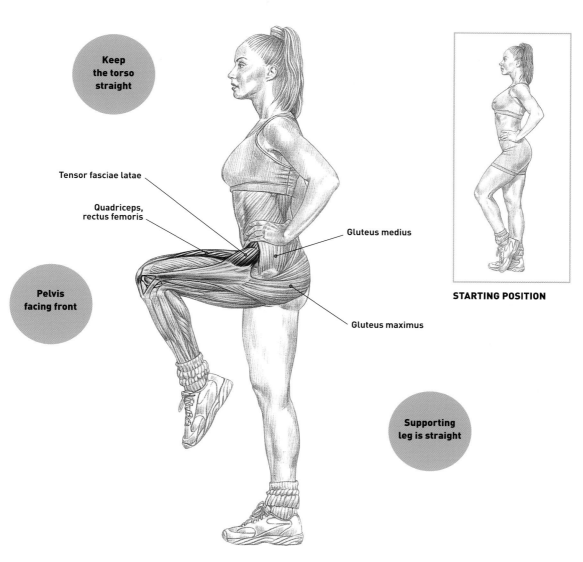

Keep the torso straight

Tensor fasciae latae

Quadriceps, rectus femoris

Gluteus medius

Pelvis facing front

Gluteus maximus

Supporting leg is straight

STARTING POSITION

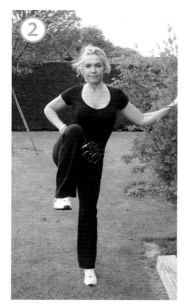

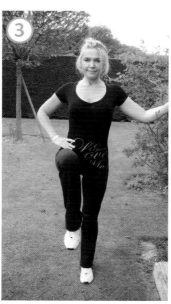

Body-Weight Squat

Targets Works the quadriceps and the buttocks. This is a complete exercise for the lower body as well as an excellent warm-up. It is also a good exercise if you are a beginner because it will help you learn the bending movement used in the squat (see pages 112-113).

Repetitions Do 4 sets of 30 repetitions.

Your coach's advice If you have trouble doing this exercise without falling forward, you may have stiff ankles or long femurs (the upper bone of the leg). To remedy this problem, put a small wedge (such as a yoga mat folded in thirds) under your heels, but be careful to keep your balance.

Breathing Inhale as you go down and exhale as you come up.

Warning Keep your chest out and your back straight but not arched. Do not round your back. Do not lean your head forward; keep it in line with your spine.

Key to the exercise To make this exercise most effective, you must control your descent and perform the exercise without jerky motions. Your back should be very straight and your heels should never leave the floor.

1. Stand with your legs slightly apart, arms straight in front of you or down at your sides, head and back very straight, and chest open. Inhale as you bend your legs. Once you have lowered your body down, your thighs should be parallel to the floor.

2. Exhale as you stand up and return to the starting position.

3. Repeat until you have completed the set.

Variation To make this exercise more intense, you can stay in the bent-knee position for 4 or 5 seconds. Holding your arms out in front of you will help you maintain your posture without falling forward and will also help you tone the underside of your arms at the same time. You can also do this exercise with your arms crossed in front of you or held at your sides.

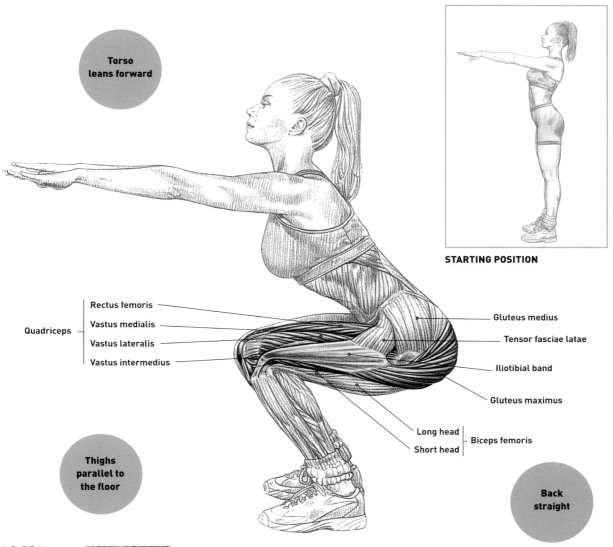

Torso leans forward

STARTING POSITION

Quadriceps
- Rectus femoris
- Vastus medialis
- Vastus lateralis
- Vastus intermedius

Gluteus medius

Tensor fasciae latae

Iliotibial band

Gluteus maximus

Long head — Biceps femoris
Short head

Thighs parallel to the floor

Back straight

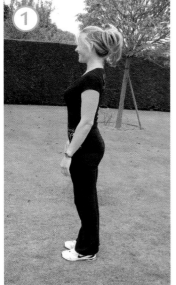

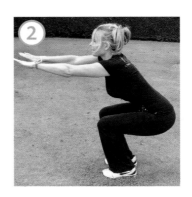

VARIATIONS: arms crossed in front or held at the sides

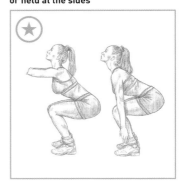

Deadlift

Targets Works your quadriceps, adductors, and gluteus maximus. If you use a weight, you will also engage your trapezius muscles, not to mention the lower back muscles.

Repetitions Do 4 sets of 15 repetitions.

Your coach's advice You can start out doing the exercise with just a bar until you are certain you can perform the exercise correctly and that you are not at risk of injuring yourself. After that, add a small amount of weight (15 to 25 pounds, or about 7 to 11 kg).

Breathing Inhale as you go down and exhale as you come up.

Warning If you perform this exercise incorrectly, you could injure your lower back. Keep both arms straight, contract your buttocks muscles, and tighten your abdominal muscles so that you do not hurt your back.

Key to the exercise Be sure that your shoes are tight enough to give your ankles good support.

1. Stand with your legs apart and your feet parallel or turned out. Always keep your feet in line with your knees. Bend your legs to bring your thighs to a horizontal position.

2. Lean your torso slightly forward and engage your abdominal and buttocks muscles. Grab a bar off the floor with both palms facing you or one hand pronated (palm facing you) and the other supinated (palm facing out) to keep the bar from sliding, depending on the weight you are using.

3. Exhale as you stand up. Do not make any jerky movements, and keep your back straight and your abdominal and buttocks muscles engaged throughout. Inhale as you set the bar down.

Variation Depending on the position of your feet and the width of your legs, you can work your back muscles or your quadriceps to a greater or lesser degree. You can change the amount of weight you lift, but be careful not to overestimate your own strength!

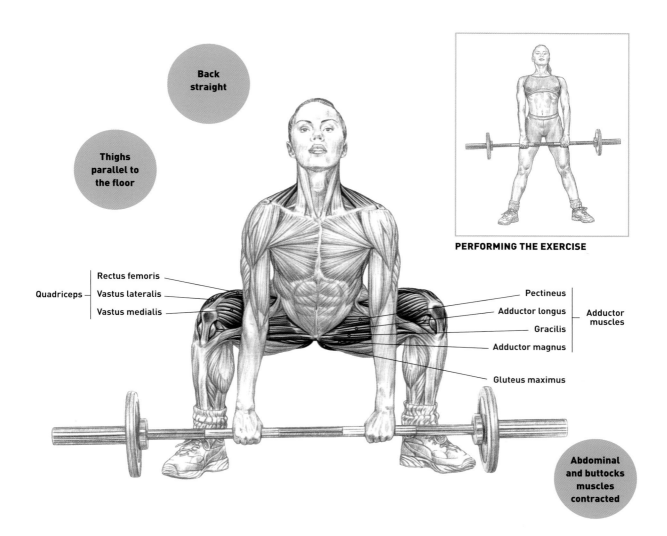

Back straight

Thighs parallel to the floor

PERFORMING THE EXERCISE

Quadriceps — Rectus femoris

Vastus lateralis

Vastus medialis

Pectineus

Adductor longus

Gracilis

Adductor magnus

Adductor muscles

Gluteus maximus

Abdominal and buttocks muscles contracted

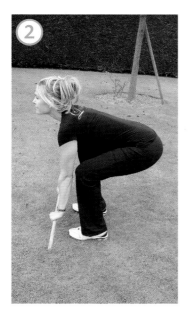

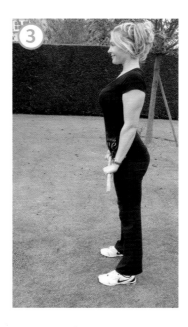

Squat With a Bar

Targets   This two-in-one exercise tones the thighs and the buttocks.

Repetitions   Do 4 sets of 15 repetitions.

Your coach's advice   Be sure to keep your torso straight. To prevent injury to your lower back, never round your back. Tighten your abdominal muscles and contract your buttocks when you go down and when you come up.

Breathing   Exhale as you come up and inhale as you go down.

Warning   To avoid injury to your knees, position your feet correctly. They should be about shoulder-width apart and either parallel or slightly turned out (do what feels most natural for you).

Key to the exercise   Go down as far as you can without lifting your heels off the floor or rounding your back. You must execute both the downward and the upward movements with control so that you do them correctly and gradually.

① Stand with your legs apart and feet parallel, and place a bar just above your shoulders so that you can keep your back very straight. Open your chest and keep your back straight.

② As you inhale, bend your legs to a right angle and lean your torso slightly forward. You can even go a little lower so long as you do not round your back or pull your heels off the floor.

③ As you exhale, come back up, tightening your abdominal muscles and contracting your buttocks. Repeat until you complete the set.

Variation   To make this exercise more intense, you can hold the bent-leg position for 4 or 5 seconds before you come back up. Also, squats with a bar can be a good introduction to weighted squats. If you are confident and performing the exercise correctly, you can begin using light weights (10 to 15 pounds, or about 5 to 7 kg).

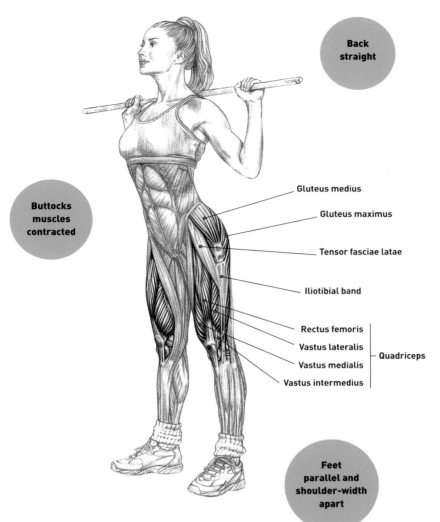

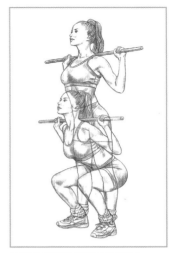

Back straight

Buttocks muscles contracted

Gluteus medius

Gluteus maximus

Tensor fasciae latae

Iliotibial band

Rectus femoris

Vastus lateralis — Quadriceps

Vastus medialis

Vastus intermedius

Feet parallel and shoulder-width apart

PERFORMING THE EXERCISE

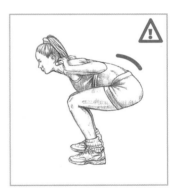

PERFORMING THE EXERCISE INCORRECTLY

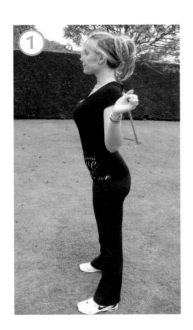

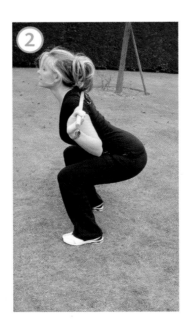

Wide-Leg Squat

Targets   In addition to the gluteus maximus, this exercise especially recruits the inner thigh muscles (adductors).

Repetitions   Do 4 sets of 15 repetitions.

Your coach's advice   The squat is one of the most complete exercises available. When done with a light weight, it will recruit the quadriceps (front of the thigh), all the adductors, the pectineus and gracilis (inner thigh), the buttocks, the hamstrings (back of the thigh), the abdominal muscles, and all the sacrolumbar muscles (lower back).

Breathing   Exhale as you come up and inhale as you go down.

Warning   Bend your knees as you lean your torso slightly forward so that you do not engage your lumbar muscles and you protect your knees.

Key to the exercise   Depending on where you place your feet, you will change the muscles that are recruited. Focus on the part of the thigh that you want to work the most.

1. Stand with your legs apart and your feet turned out. Place a stick or a slightly weighted bar above your shoulders so you can keep your back very straight. Open your chest and keep your back straight.

2. As you inhale, bend your legs and bring your thighs parallel to the floor as you lean your torso slightly forward. (Note: As you bend your legs more, you will not lean your torso as far forward.)

3. As you exhale, come up while tightening your abdominal muscles and contracting your buttocks. Repeat the exercise until you complete the set.

Variation   To make this exercise more intense, you can hold the bent-leg position for 4 or 5 seconds before you come up. You can also vary the weight you use, from 10 to 15 pounds (about 5 to 7 kg). Finally, do not forget that depending on where you place your feet, you will focus the work on different muscles.

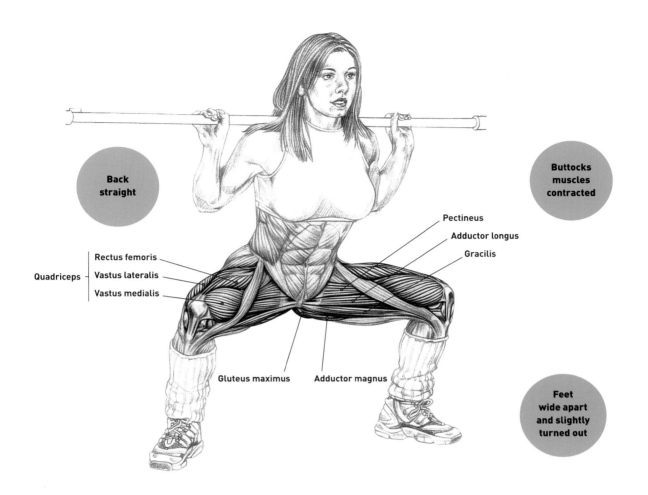

Back straight

Buttocks muscles contracted

Pectineus

Adductor longus

Gracilis

Quadriceps
Rectus femoris
Vastus lateralis
Vastus medialis

Gluteus maximus   Adductor magnus

Feet wide apart and slightly turned out

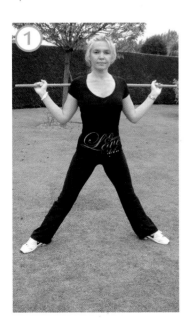

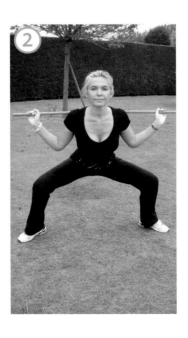

VARIATION: three ways to place the feet during a squat

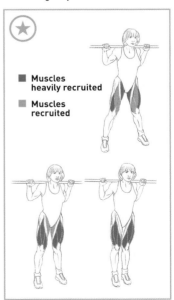

Muscles heavily recruited

Muscles recruited

Good Morning With a Bar

Targets   This exercise delicately strengthens your buttocks and develops good posture.

Repetitions   Do 3 sets of 20 repetitions.

Your coach's advice   This exercise will help you stretch and strengthen all the muscles in your back as well as give you beautiful posture. It is also ideal for strengthening the buttocks delicately, because it strengthens the muscles while stretching them.

Breathing   Inhale as you go down and exhale as you come up.

Warning   Do not arch your back, and keep your head in line with your spine. You should not round your back, either, because you could compress your vertebrae.

Key to the exercise   To make this exercise truly effective, do each repetition slowly and focus on your muscle sensations.

1. Stand with your feet parallel and hip-width apart. Place a bar on your shoulder blades to keep your back straight.

2. Inhale and lean your torso forward without arching or rounding your back. Lower until your torso is perpendicular to the floor.

3. Exhale as you come back up gradually while contracting your buttocks.

★ **Variation**   You can do this exercise with slightly bent knees as you go down. This will allow you to control the curve of your back, but it will not work your hamstrings as much.

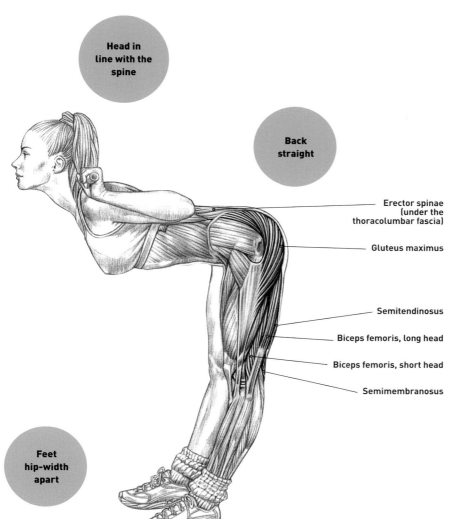

Head in line with the spine

Back straight

Erector spinae (under the thoracolumbar fascia)

Gluteus maximus

Semitendinosus

Biceps femoris, long head

Biceps femoris, short head

Semimembranosus

Feet hip-width apart

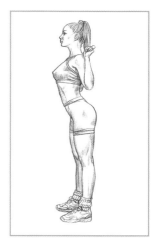

STARTING POSITION

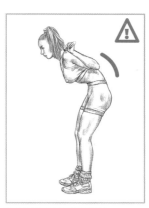

INCORRECT STARTING POSITION

VARIATION: going down with slightly bent knees

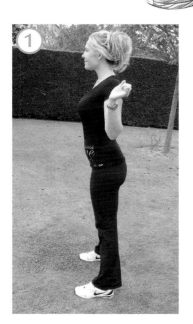

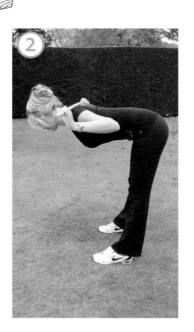

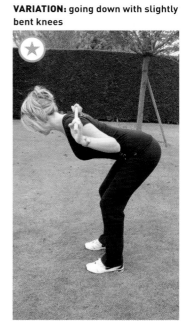

Step-Up on a Bench

Targets   Works the gluteus maximus (for a nicely toned butt) and the quadriceps (front of the thigh).

Repetitions   Do 3 or 4 sets of 20 to 30 repetitions on each leg.

Your coach's advice   To optimize your workout, synchronize your breathing with the up-and-down movements. You will see that this creates a dynamic that will encourage you during the exercise.

Breathing   Exhale as you go up and inhale as you go down.

Warning   Keeping your arms crossed in front of your chest will help you focus more on your buttocks without contracting your back too much. Be sure not to arch your back; keep it very straight.

Key to the exercise   Once on the bench, you can raise your back leg a little higher, which will accentuate the work of the buttocks muscle.

① Stand with one foot flat on the floor and your arms crossed in front of your chest (however, they should not be touching your chest). Bend your other leg and place your foot on the bench.

② Inhale and then, as you exhale, step up on the bench with the other leg held slightly behind you to maintain your balance. Tighten your abdominals and contract your buttocks muscles.

③ Lower yourself down as you inhale, and place the sole of your foot flat on the floor. Repeat this movement about 20 times without stopping before switching sides.

⭐ **Variation**   If you have trouble keeping your back straight or you have balance problems, you can do this exercise with a stick on your shoulder blades. This variation immobilizes your arms; as a result, the leg work is more intense. You can first work one leg and then the other, or you can alternate sides within the same set.

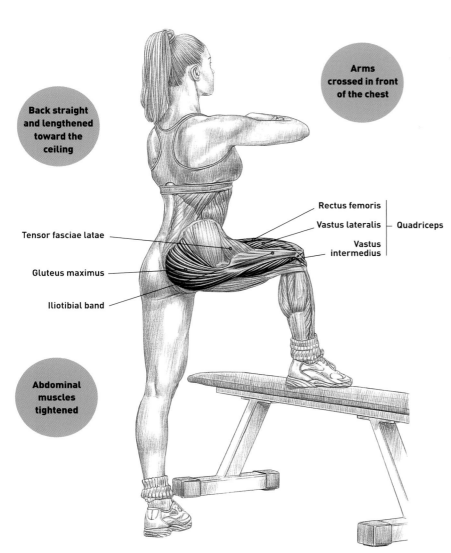

Back straight and lengthened toward the ceiling

Arms crossed in front of the chest

Tensor fasciae latae

Rectus femoris

Vastus lateralis — Quadriceps

Vastus intermedius

Gluteus maximus

Iliotibial band

Abdominal muscles tightened

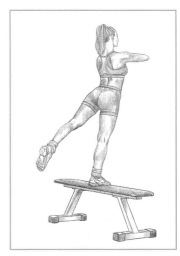

PERFORMING THE EXERCISE

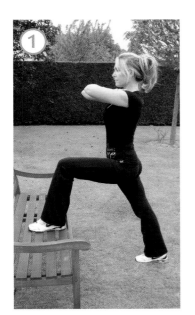

VARIATION: using a stick

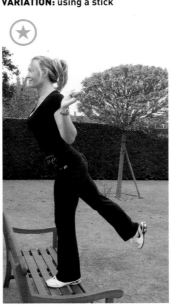

VARIATION: performing the exercise

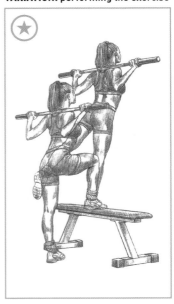

Forward Lunge

Targets To achieve nicely shaped thighs (quadriceps) and buttocks. This exercise also provides good cardiorespiratory work.

Repetitions Do 3 or 4 sets of 15 to 20 repetitions on each leg.

Your coach's advice You can alter the distance between your legs depending on which muscles you want to work. The greater the distance between your feet, the more your gluteus maximus will work; the smaller the distance, the more your quadriceps will work.

Breathing Inhale as you bend your legs and exhale as you come up.

Warning Be careful to keep your knee directly above your toes to avoid injuring your knee joint.

Key to the exercise Keep your torso very straight to get a good stretch in the quadriceps of your back leg and to tone the opposite buttock.

1. Stand with your torso straight and legs together. Place your hands on your hips.

2. Inhale and lunge forward without touching your back knee to the floor.

3. As you exhale, return to the starting position. Do a complete set on one leg and then switch legs.

Variation If you have trouble keeping your back straight or you have balance problems, you can hold your arms out in front of you. You can also start with your legs already apart and slightly bent. In this case, the exercise will consist of only bending and straightening your legs (stationary lunge). Finally, you can work one leg and then the other, or you can alternate legs within the same set. However, you will achieve better results by working each leg separately.

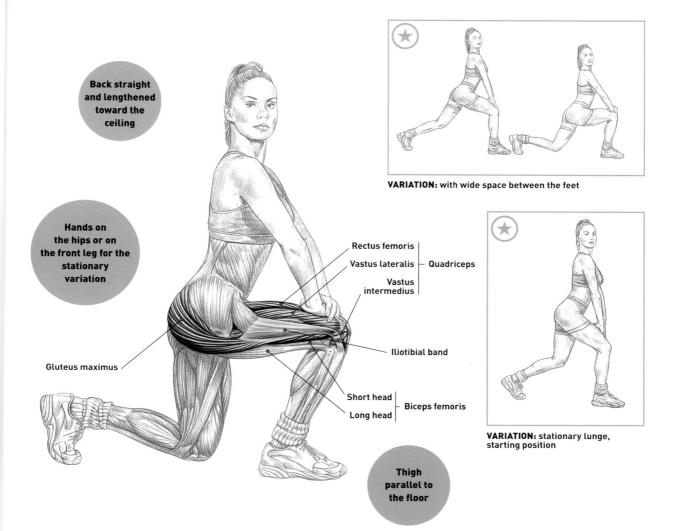

Back straight and lengthened toward the ceiling

Hands on the hips or on the front leg for the stationary variation

Gluteus maximus

Rectus femoris

Vastus lateralis — Quadriceps

Vastus intermedius

Iliotibial band

Short head

Long head — Biceps femoris

Thigh parallel to the floor

VARIATION: with wide space between the feet

VARIATION: stationary lunge, starting position

VARIATION: straight arms

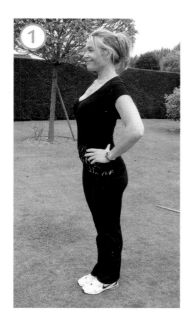

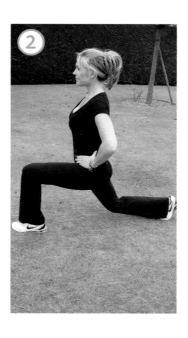

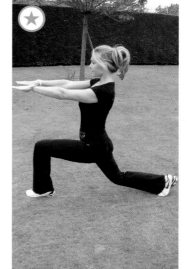

Forward Lunge With Dumbbells

Targets   Works the gluteus maximus and quadriceps muscles as well as the arms (statically).

Repetitions   Do 3 or 4 sets of 15 to 20 repetitions on each leg.

Your coach's advice   Because you feel most of the weight as you bend the leg and this exercise also requires good balance to protect the knee joint, you should start with a light weight.

Breathing   Inhale as you bend your legs and exhale as you come back up.

Warning   Do not arch your back and be sure to engage your abdominal wall. At the end of the bending movement, your front knee should be directly over your ankle. Do not let your knee go past your ankle.

Key to the exercise   If you want to work the gluteus maximus, take a large step forward. If you prefer to work the quadriceps, then take a small step forward. Go down slowly, with control; once your thigh is horizontal, use your muscles to push up and return to the starting position.

(1) Stand with your torso straight, legs straight, arms at your sides, and dumbbells in hands.

(2) As you exhale, take a large step forward and keep your torso as straight as possible.

(3) As you inhale, return to the starting position, moving your body energetically. Do an entire set on the same leg and then switch legs.

Variation   You can work one leg and then the other or you can alternate legs within the same set. However, you will achieve better results if you work the legs separately. You can also alternate between forward and backward lunges by putting one leg behind you and simultaneously leaning your torso with your arms at your sides. This will let you synergistically work all the muscles in the butt and thigh as well as the arms.

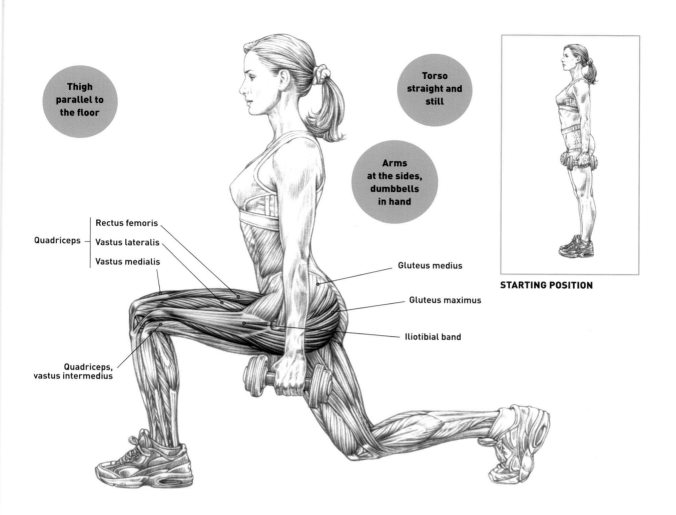

Thigh
parallel to
the floor

Torso
straight and
still

Arms
at the sides,
dumbbells
in hand

Quadriceps
- Rectus femoris
- Vastus lateralis
- Vastus medialis

Gluteus medius

Gluteus maximus

Iliotibial band

Quadriceps,
vastus intermedius

STARTING POSITION

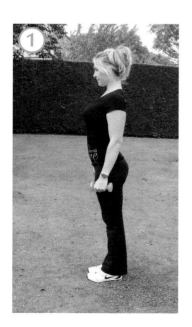

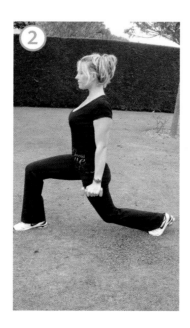

Alternating Side Lunge

◎ **Targets**   Works all the quadriceps muscles and the gluteus medius and gluteus maximus (front of the thighs as well as the side and back part of the buttock) of the bent leg. Also stretches the adductor muscles of the straight leg.

Ⓛ **Repetitions**   Do 3 or 4 sets of 20 alternating repetitions.

◉◉ **Your coach's advice**   Because this exercise requires you to move a large part of your body weight to one leg, we recommend that you work in sets of 20 alternating repetitions maximum (so 10 on the right leg and 10 on the left leg). Be sure to perform the exercise correctly to protect your knees.

◉ **Breathing**   Inhale as you bend your leg and exhale as you come back up.

❗ **Warning**   To protect your knees and ankles, try to keep both soles of your feet on the floor as much as possible when you lower into the lunge.

🔑 **Key to the exercise**   Lean your torso forward as you bend your legs so that you do not engage your lower back. This will also help you focus the work on the adductor muscles of the straight leg and the outer thigh of the bent leg.

① Stand with your torso straight and legs straight (either touching or shoulder-width apart). Your arms should rest at your sides.

② As you inhale, bend one leg to the side while leaning your torso slightly forward to avoid engaging your back. Your bent knee is directly above your ankle and foot. Your thigh is parallel to the floor.

③ As you exhale, return to the starting position. Do 20 side lunges, alternating between the left and right legs.

★ **Variation**   When you are bent down, you can bring your arms in front of you (which will recruit them) or you can put your hands on your knee for greater stability. Vary your range of motion in the exercise: If your feet are close together or only slightly apart, then you will need to take a large step to the side on every lunge. For more static work, step out as wide as you want, and then simply straighten your bent leg, shifting your weight to the other side as you bend your other leg.

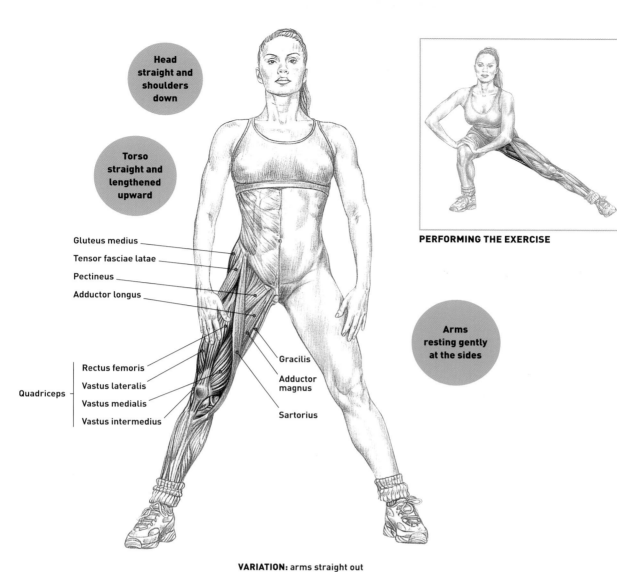

Head straight and shoulders down

Torso straight and lengthened upward

Gluteus medius

Tensor fasciae latae

Pectineus

Adductor longus

Quadriceps
- Rectus femoris
- Vastus lateralis
- Vastus medialis
- Vastus intermedius

Gracilis

Adductor magnus

Sartorius

Arms resting gently at the sides

PERFORMING THE EXERCISE

VARIATION: arms straight out

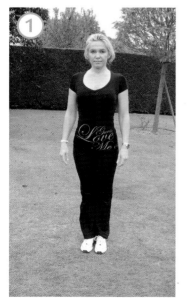

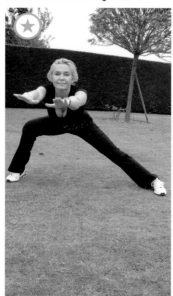

Standing Hamstring Stretch

Targets This stretch provides definition and lengthens the entire back of the leg from the gluteus maximus to the calf muscles.

Repetitions Hold the stretch for 30 to 40 seconds on each side at the end of your leg workout.

Your coach's advice Always do stretches gently and with moderation to protect your joints, and avoid overstretching your ligaments. Work with your breathing and try to stretch a little farther with each exhalation, but do not make any abrupt movements.

Breathing Inhale and exhale deeply and calmly throughout the stretch.

Warning Since most of your body weight is resting on the supporting leg, bend it slightly and rest your hands on it to relieve pressure on the knee joint.

Key to the exercise Keeping your back straight, lean your torso forward as much as you can to intensify the stretch, especially in the buttocks muscles. Flex the foot of your straight leg so you can really recruit your calf muscles.

1. Stand with your spine stretched toward the ceiling and bring one straight leg in front of you. Flex your foot and let the weight rest on the heel. Your other leg is slightly bent (the knee should not go beyond the tip of the foot), and your torso begins to lean forward.

2. Put both hands on your bent thigh and shift your torso forward, keeping your back straight to accentuate the stretch.

3. Hold the stretch and breathe deeply. Switch legs.

★ **Variation** If you are more flexible, you can stretch both legs at the same time by shifting your pelvis forward with the legs straight and squeezed together and the feet parallel. Keep both legs straight and, depending on your flexibility, place your hands behind your knees, calves, or ankles.

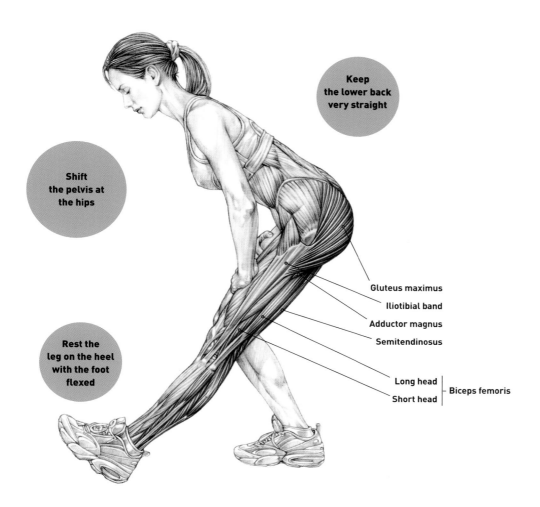

Shift the pelvis at the hips

Keep the lower back very straight

Rest the leg on the heel with the foot flexed

Gluteus maximus

Iliotibial band

Adductor magnus

Semitendinosus

Long head

Short head

Biceps femoris

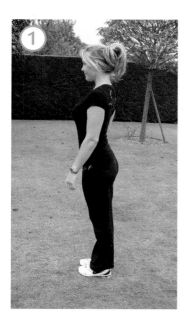

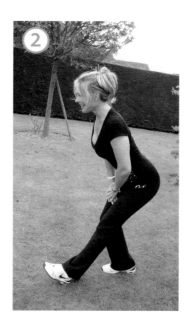

ADVANCED VARIATION

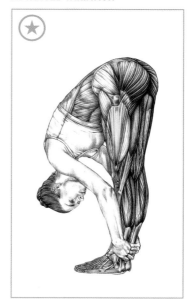

Hamstring Stretch Using a Bench

Targets   This stretch provides definition and elongates the entire back of the leg from the gluteus maximus to the calf muscles.

Repetitions   Hold the stretch for 30 to 40 seconds on each side at the end of your leg workout.

Your coach's advice   Stretching at the end of a workout is an ideal time to relax from the pressure of your day. Try to clear your mind, concentrate on your breathing, and imagine that you are letting go of any negative thoughts each time you exhale.

Breathing   Inhale and exhale deeply and calmly throughout the stretch.

Warning   Put your hands on your working leg to control the descent of your torso. Never round your back, even if it you can go down only a few inches. Your pelvis is what moves; your back does not bend.

Key to the exercise   The entire spinal column is stretched. Keep your head in line with your spine.

1. Stand with your spine lengthened toward the ceiling and put one straight leg in front of you on a bench. Flex your foot. Keep your standing leg straight and lean your torso slightly forward.

2. Place both hands on the thigh of your raised leg and lean your torso forward. Keep your back straight to accentuate the stretch.

3. Hold the stretch and breathe deeply. Switch legs.

Variation   Depending on your flexibility, you can place your leg on a support that is shorter or taller than a bench. The important thing is to keep your hips level and to initiate the movement from your pelvis. Flex the foot of your raised leg to stretch your calf muscles as well. However, if you wish to focus the stretch on the buttock and hamstring instead, then just point your foot.

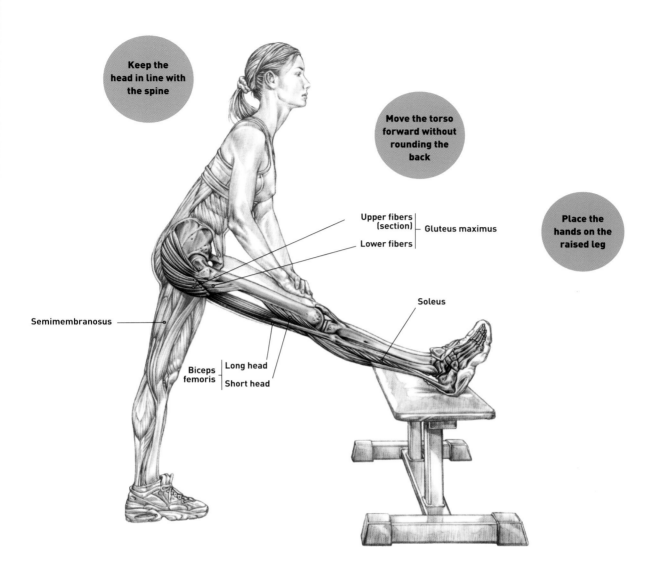

Keep the head in line with the spine

Move the torso forward without rounding the back

Place the hands on the raised leg

Upper fibers (section) — Gluteus maximus
Lower fibers

Soleus

Semimembranosus

Biceps femoris
Long head
Short head

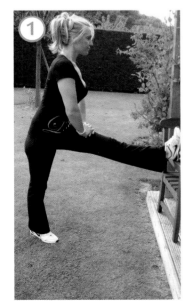

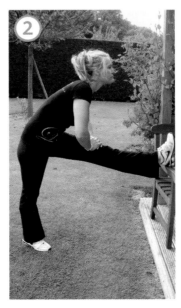

Standing Calf Raise

Targets   Works the calves to give the lower leg more definition.

Repetitions   Do 3 sets of 20 repetitions.

Your coach's advice   When done without support, this exercise forces you to work on your balance, especially by contracting the abdominal wall. Remember to go up and down slowly.

Breathing   Exhale as you go up and inhale as you go down.

Warning   Keep your torso straight, your shoulders down and back, and your pelvis tilted slightly backward (see page 30). To keep your balance, engage your abdominal and buttocks muscles.

Key to the exercise   The placement of your feet determines whether you work the outer part of the calves (feet turned in) or the inner part of the calves (feet turned out). Unless you are at an advanced level you should do parallel-feet variations only when you are working with a support.

1. Stand with your legs together and your feet parallel. Put your hands on your hips and contract your buttocks and abdominal muscles slightly.

2. As you exhale, slowly rise up onto the balls of your feet.

3. As you inhale, gradually come back down to the starting position. Repeat until you complete your set.

Variation   If you have difficulty keeping your balance, you can place both of your hands on a chair or put one hand on another support (a wall or door frame). To increase the intensity of the exercise and stretch the muscles on the soles of the feet as you go down, you can do this exercise on a stair or step. But for that variation, you must absolutely hold on to a support of some kind.

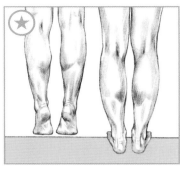

VARIATION: performing the exercise on a step

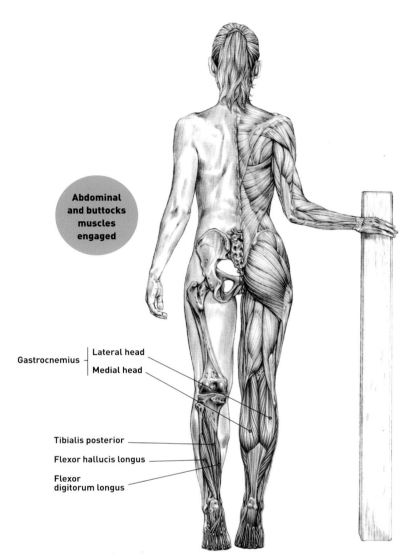

Abdominal and buttocks muscles engaged

Gastrocnemius — Lateral head
Medial head

Tibialis posterior

Flexor hallucis longus

Flexor digitorum longus

Legs straight and parallel

Stretching and relaxing the feet gradually

VARIATION: hands resting on a chair

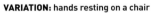

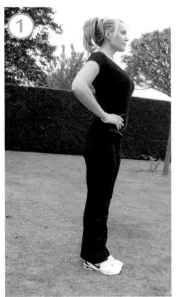

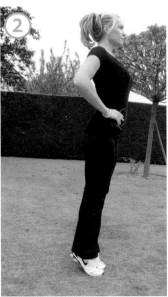

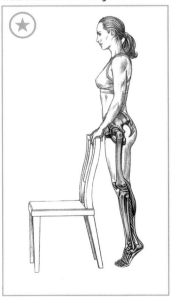

131

Calf Raise Using a Dumbbell

Targets   Works the calves in isolation to sculpt the lower part of the leg.

Repetitions   Do 3 or 4 sets of 20 to 30 repetitions.

Your coach's advice   This exercise works one calf at a time. Because it is effective in long sets (until you feel a burning sensation in the calf), you should do it one side at a time, without alternating legs.

Breathing   Exhale as you go up and inhale as you come down.

Warning   Your torso should be straight, abdominal wall engaged, and buttocks tightened so that you do not compensate with your lower back or put too much weight on your joints.

Key to the exercise   To make this exercise more effective, focus on contracting your buttocks when you go up and when you come down. Also, it will not help to use heavy weights; a small dumbbell will suffice.

1. Stand on your right leg with the front of your foot on a step or stair and bend your other leg slightly. Hold on to a support with your left hand to keep from losing your balance. Grab a dumbbell with your right hand, keeping that arm down at your side.

2. As you exhale, rise up slowly onto the ball of the right foot.

3. As you exhale, gradually return to the starting position and even go a little beyond (heel hanging in the air and lower than the ball of your right foot). Repeat until your set is complete. Switch legs.

Variation   Once you have mastered this exercise, you can hold the raised position for 4 or 5 seconds, stop midway through your descent and hold that position for 4 or 5 seconds, and hold the lower position for 4 or 5 seconds before returning to the starting position.

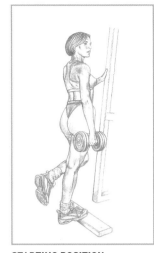

STARTING POSITION

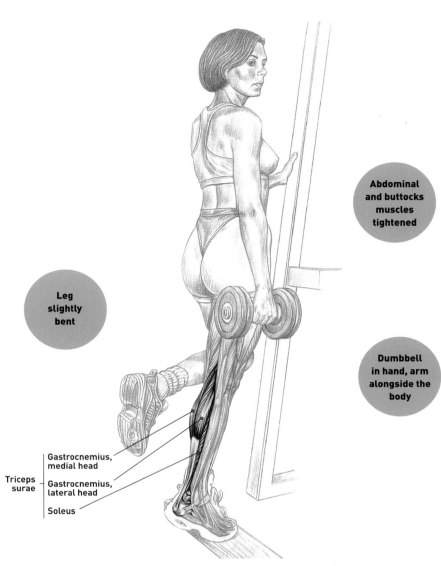

Abdominal and buttocks muscles tightened

Leg slightly bent

Dumbbell in hand, arm alongside the body

Triceps surae
Gastrocnemius, medial head
Gastrocnemius, lateral head
Soleus

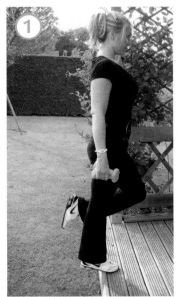

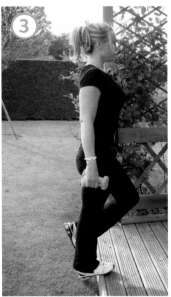

Calf Stretch

◎ **Targets**   This stretch provides definition and elongates the entire lower leg.

🕐 **Repetitions**   Hold the stretch for 30 to 40 seconds on each side after your calf and leg workout.

👓 **Your coach's advice**   This exercise is very effective for stretching the calves at the end of a leg workout, but it is also helpful if you need to get rid of leg cramps at any time during the day or during a workout.

😮 **Breathing**   Inhale and exhale deeply and calmly throughout the stretch.

❗ **Warning**   Your pelvis faces front, your hips are level, and your back is straight and leaning slightly forward. The knee of your bent leg should never go beyond the tip of your foot.

🔑 **Key to the exercise**   This stretch is effective only if you keep both heels on the floor.

1 Stand with your spine lengthened toward the ceiling and hands on your hips. Put one leg forward with the foot flat on the floor. Both legs should be straight and your torso should lean slightly forward.

2 Gradually bend the knee of your forward leg and bring the knee directly over your ankle. Your pelvis moves forward and your back leg stays straight. Both of your heels should stay firmly on the floor.

3 Hold the stretch and breathe deeply. Switch legs.

⭐ **Variation**   To make this stretch even better, you can do it facing a wall. Put both palms flat on the wall and push the wall as you do the forward bending movement. Depending on your flexibility, you can also put your bent leg on a support (bench or low wall) to stretch your adductors at the same time.

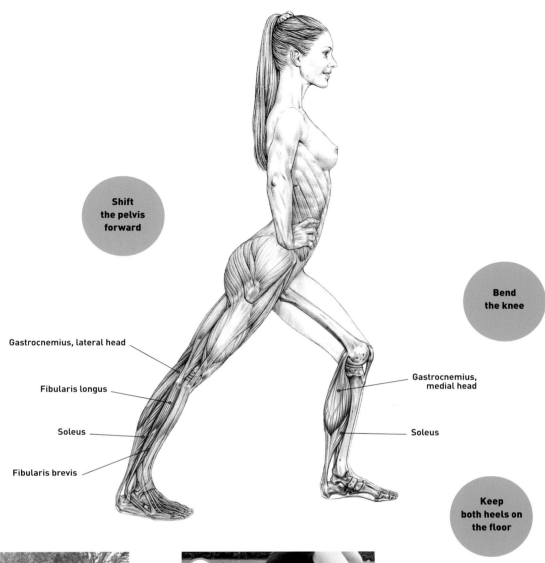

Shift the pelvis forward

Bend the knee

Keep both heels on the floor

Gastrocnemius, lateral head

Fibularis longus

Soleus

Fibularis brevis

Gastrocnemius, medial head

Soleus

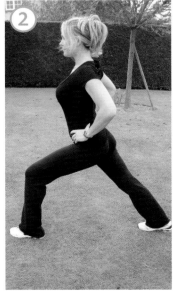

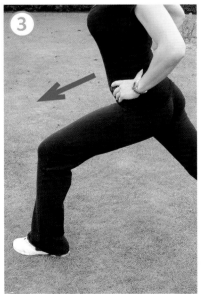

Develop Your Own
CUSTOMIZED PROGRAM

DOMINANT CHARACTERISTICS

· ·

When observing people around you, you have undoubtedly noticed that they can generally be classified into one of three broad physical categories.

These three morphological classifications arise from the development of the embryo. Beginning in the second week of embryonic development, there are three primitive layers: the external layer, called the ectoderm; the middle layer, called the mesoderm; and the deep layer, called the endoderm.

Each of these layers is the origin of what will later become very specific parts of the organism:

→ The ectoderm will form the epidermis and sensory organs, the central nervous system, and the peripheral nerves.

→ The mesoderm will primarily form the bones, muscles, urogenital organs, circulatory system, and blood.

→ The endoderm, finally, will form the intestinal mucosa and auxiliary glands.

Ⓐ ECTOMORPH

Ectomorphs are usually thin and have narrow shoulders. They have very active metabolisms and almost no body fat; however, they often lack muscle tone, which causes back problems, poor posture, and a prominent belly.

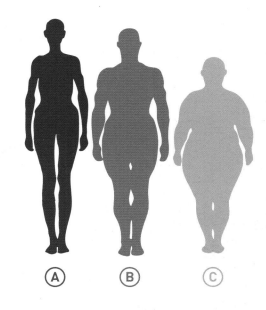

Ⓐ   Ⓑ   Ⓒ

Ectomorphic women must therefore focus on developing postural muscles and deep abdominal muscles.

Ⓑ MESOMORPH

Mesomorphs are generally muscular and toned with thick bones and joints, wide shoulders, and well-developed rib cages.

Generally, people with this body type are not too stout, and a minimum amount of physical training will produce a maximum result.

Also, mesomorphs typically are very active, so they enjoy moving and participating in sports.

C ENDOMORPH

Endomorphs are characterized by their curves, which often hide their bones and muscles. The skeleton of an endomorph is not as massive as that of a mesomorph, but a slower metabolism means they have a tendency to gain weight, especially in the thighs and waist, which can lead to knee problems.

To stay in shape and maintain a healthy weight, endomorphs need to do regular physical activity and avoid overtraining; they also need to avoid high-calorie, low-nutrient diets.

PERSONALIZING YOUR TRAINING

These morphology types are extremes; that is, it's rare to encounter a pure ectomorph or a pure endomorph in nature. Most people have a mixed morphology. But it is important to learn to recognize the major traits of your physical nature, because you cannot change your predominant type. However, you can work on your weak areas to refine the things you do not like.

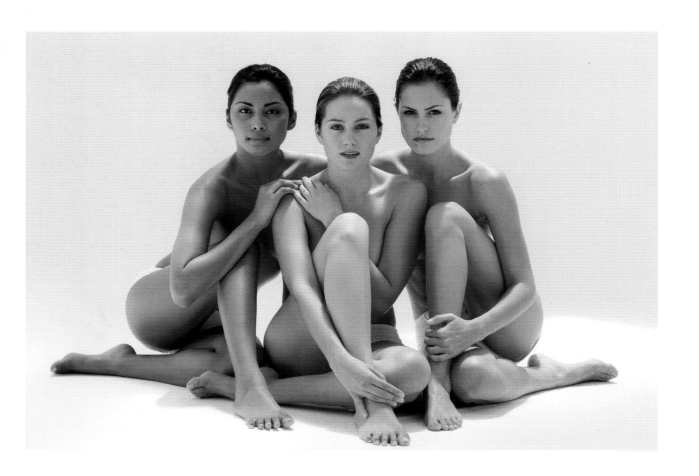

DESIGN YOUR PROGRAM

Once you understand these basic concepts of anatomy, you will be able to design a custom program that will give you more definition and tone so that you can get the body you've always wanted.

First, you must do the following:

1. Define your basic morphology: A (ecto-morph), B (mesomorph), or C (endomorph).
2. Devote yourself to your workout program 2 to 3 hours per week.
3. Hydrate your body before, during, and after workouts.
4. Integrate 5 to 10 minutes of stretching into each workout.

→ MORPHOLOGY A

PROGRAM 1 **BEGINNER**

GOAL 1: SLIM YOUR WAIST AND STRETCH YOUR BODY

❑ **Torso twist with a stick** (→ p. 42),
2 sets of 30 reps

❑ **Static stretch for the waist** (→ p. 38),
2 sets of 30 seconds

GOAL 2: STRENGTHEN AND TONE YOUR ABDOMINALS

❑ **Bicycle** (→ p. 68), 2 sets of 15 reps

❑ **Leg extension** (→ p. 64), 3 sets of 20 reps

❑ **Crunch, feet on the floor** (→ p. 52),
3 sets of 15 reps

GOAL 3: STRENGTHEN AND SHAPE YOUR BUTTOCKS

❑ **Leg lift to the side** (→ p. 76),
2 sets of 15 reps on each leg

❑ **Opposite arm and leg raise** (→ p. 84),
2 sets of 30 seconds on each side

❑ **Bridge** (→ p. 88), 3 sets of 20 reps

❑ **Leg extension to the side** (→ p. 100),
2 sets of 20 reps on each leg

GOAL 4: STRENGTHEN AND SHAPE YOUR LEGS

❑ **Body-weight squat** (→ p. 108),
2 sets of 10 reps

❑ **Wide-leg squat** (→ p. 114),
2 sets of 10 reps

❑ **Step-up on a bench** (→ p. 118),
1 set of 10 reps on each leg

❑ **Calf raise using a dumbbell** (→ p. 132),
2 sets of 15 reps on each leg

PROGRAM 2 **INTERMEDIATE**

GOAL 1: SLIM YOUR WAIST AND STRETCH YOUR BODY

❑ **Static stretch for the waist** (→ p. 38),
2 or 3 sets, 40 seconds each

❑ **Hamstring stretch using a bench** (→ p. 128),
2 sets of 1 minute on each leg

❑ **Sphinx** (→ p. 72), 2 sets of 1 to 2 minutes each

GOAL 2: STRENGTHEN AND TONE YOUR ABDOMINALS

❑ **Sit-up, feet on the floor** (→ p. 56),
3 sets of 20 reps

❑ **Crunch, feet on a bench** (→ p. 58),
3 sets of 20 reps

❑ **Reverse crunch** (→ p. 66), 3 sets of 20 reps

❑ **Crunch, legs raised** (→ p. 54), 3 sets of 30 reps

GOAL 3: STRENGTHEN AND SHAPE YOUR BUTTOCKS

- ❑ **Leg lift on the knees** (➔ p. 80),
  2 sets of 30 reps on each leg

- ❑ **Bridge, feet on a bench** (➔ p. 90),
  3 sets of 20 reps

- ❑ **Bridge, one leg raised** (➔ p. 92),
  3 sets of 20 reps on each leg

- ❑ **Side leg raise on the knees** (➔ p. 86),
  3 sets of 20 reps on each leg

GOAL 4: STRENGTHEN AND SHAPE YOUR LEGS

- ❑ **Squat with a bar** (➔ p. 112), 3 sets of 20 reps

- ❑ **Wide-leg squat** (➔ p. 114), 3 sets of 20 reps

- ❑ **Forward lunge** (➔ p. 120),
  3 sets of 15 reps on each leg

- ❑ **Alternating side lunge** (➔ p. 124),
  2 sets of 20 reps on each side

PROGRAM 3 **ADVANCED**

GOAL 1: STRETCH YOUR BODY

- ❑ **Buttocks stretch** (➔ p. 96),
  3 sets of 2 minutes on each leg

- ❑ **Lying hamstring stretch** (➔ p. 94),
  2 sets of 3 minutes on each leg

- ❑ **Sphinx** (➔ p. 72), 2 sets of 3 minutes

GOAL 2: STRENGTHEN AND TONE YOUR ABDOMINALS

- ❑ **Crunch, legs raised** (➔ p. 54),
  4 sets of 30 reps

- ❑ **Oblique crunch, legs raised** (➔ p. 62),
  3 sets of 30 reps

- ❑ **Oblique bicycle** (➔ p. 70), 4 sets of 30 reps

- ❑ **Reverse crunch** (➔ p. 66), 3 sets of 40 reps

GOAL 3: STRENGTHEN AND SHAPE YOUR BUTTOCKS

- ❑ **Leg lift with a bent knee** (➔ p. 82),
  4 sets of 30 reps on each leg

- ❑ **Side leg raise on the knees** (➔ p. 86),
  4 sets of 30 reps on each leg

- ❑ **Bridge, one leg raised** (➔ p. 92),
  4 sets of 20 reps on each leg using a 2 lb. (1 kg)
  weight

- ❑ **Lateral leg curl** (➔ p. 102), 3 sets of 30 reps
  on each leg using a 2 lb. (1 kg) weight

GOAL 4: STRENGTHEN AND SHAPE YOUR LEGS

- ❑ **Deadlift** (➔ p. 110), 3 sets of 30 reps

- ❑ **Good morning with a bar** (➔ p. 116),
  4 sets of 20 reps with a 10 to 15 lb. (5 to 7 kg)
  bar

- ❑ **Forward lunge with dumbbells** (➔ p. 122),
  4 sets of 20 reps on each leg with a 10 lb. (5 kg)
  weight in each hand

- ❑ **Step-up on a bench** (➔ p. 118),
  3 sets of 20 reps on each leg

➔ MORPHOLOGY **B**

PROGRAM 1 **BEGINNER**

GOAL 1: SLIM YOUR WAIST AND STRETCH YOUR BODY

- ❑ **Buttocks stretch** (➔ p. 96),
  2 sets of 30 seconds on each leg

- ❑ **Calf stretch** (➔ p. 134), 2 sets of 30 seconds
  on each leg

- ❑ **Lying torso twist** (➔ p. 44),
  2 sets of 30 seconds on each side

GOAL 2: STRENGTHEN AND TONE YOUR ABDOMINALS

- ❑ **Sit-up, feet on the floor** (➔ p. 56),
  3 sets of 15 reps

- ❑ **Crunch, feet on a bench** (➔ p. 58),
  3 sets of 15 reps

- ❑ **Oblique crunch, legs raised** (➔ p. 62),
  4 sets of 10 reps

❑ **Leg extension** (→ p. 64), 4 sets of 20 reps

GOAL 3: STRENGTHEN AND SHAPE YOUR BUTTOCKS

❑ **Leg lift to the side** (→ p. 76),
3 sets of 30 reps on each leg

❑ **Leg extension to the back** (→ p. 98),
4 sets of 30 reps on each leg

❑ **Leg extension to the side** (→ p. 100),
3 sets of 30 reps on each leg

❑ **Bridge** (→ p. 88), 3 sets of 20 reps

GOAL 4: STRENGTHEN AND SHAPE YOUR LEGS

❑ **Standing knee raise** (→ p. 106),
3 sets of 20 reps on each leg

❑ **Squat with a bar** (→ p. 112),
2 sets of 20 reps

❑ **Good morning with a bar** (→ p. 116),
3 sets of 20 reps

❑ **Standing calf raise** (→ p. 130),
4 sets of 30 reps

PROGRAM 2 **INTERMEDIATE**

GOAL 1: SLIM YOUR WAIST AND STRETCH YOUR BODY

❑ **Sphinx** (→ p. 72), 2 sets of 30 to 40 seconds

❑ **Buttocks stretch** (→ p. 96),
2 sets of 1 minute on each leg

❑ **Lying hamstring stretch** (→ p. 94),
3 sets of 1 minute on each leg

GOAL 2: STRENGTHEN AND TONE YOUR ABDOMINALS

❑ **Crunch, legs raised** (→ p. 54),
4 sets of 30 reps

❑ **Oblique bicycle** (→ p. 70), 4 sets of 30 reps

❑ **Crunch, feet on a bench** (→ p. 58),
4 or 5 sets of 30 reps

❑ **Reverse crunch** (→ p. 66), 5 sets of 30 reps

❑ **Oblique crunch, legs raised** (→ p. 62),
3 sets of 20 reps

GOAL 3: STRENGTHEN AND SHAPE YOUR BUTTOCKS

❑ **Leg lift to the side** (→ p. 76),
4 sets of 15 reps on each leg

❑ **Leg lift on the knees** (→ p. 80),
4 sets of 30 reps on each leg

❑ **Bridge** (→ p. 88), 3 sets of 30 reps

GOAL 4: STRENGTHEN AND SHAPE YOUR LEGS

❑ **Forward lunge** (→ p. 120),
3 sets of 20 reps on each leg

❑ **Step-up on a bench** (→ p. 118),
3 sets of 20 reps on each leg

❑ **Alternating side lunge** (→ p. 124),
3 sets of 15 reps on each side

❑ **Squat with a bar** (→ p. 112), 5 sets of 20 reps

PROGRAM 3 **ADVANCED**

GOAL 1: SLIM YOUR WAIST AND STRETCH YOUR BODY

❑ **Standing side bend** (→ p. 40),
4 sets of 20 reps on each side

❑ **Side plank** (→ p. 46), 4 sets of 40 reps
on each side

❑ **Standing hamstring stretch** (→ p. 126),
3 sets of 30 to 40 seconds on each leg

❑ **Hamstring stretch using a bench** (→ p. 128),
3 sets of 1 minute on each leg

❑ **Static stretch for the waist** (→ p. 38),
2 sets of 30 seconds

GOAL 2: STRENGTHEN AND TONE YOUR ABDOMINALS

❑ **Oblique bicycle** (→ p. 70),
5 sets of 30 reps

❑ **Bicycle** (→ p. 68), 4 sets of 40 reps

- ❑ **Crunch, legs raised** (→ p. 54), 5 sets of 30 reps
- ❑ **Crunch, feet on a bench** (→ p. 58), 4 sets of 30 reps

GOAL 3: STRENGTHEN AND SHAPE YOUR BUTTOCKS

- ❑ **Bridge, feet on a bench** (→ p. 90), 4 sets of 30 reps
- ❑ **Leg lift with a bent knee** (→ p. 82), 4 sets of 20 reps on each leg
- ❑ **Side leg raise on the knees** (→ p. 86), 4 sets of 30 reps on each leg
- ❑ **Bridge with one leg raised** (→ p. 92), 3 sets of 40 reps on each leg

GOAL 4: STRENGTHEN AND SHAPE YOUR LEGS

- ❑ **Forward lunge with dumbbells** (→ p. 122), 4 sets of 30 reps on each leg
- ❑ **Step-up on a bench** (→ p. 118), 5 sets of 30 reps on each leg
- ❑ **Deadlift** (→ p. 110), 5 sets of 20 reps
- ❑ **Squat with a bar** (→ p. 112), 4 sets of 20 reps

→ MORPHOLOGY C

PROGRAM 1 **BEGINNER**

GOAL 1: STRETCH YOUR BODY

- ❑ **Lying hamstring stretch** (→ p. 94), 2 sets of 30 seconds on each leg
- ❑ **Standing hamstring stretch** (→ p. 126), 2 sets of 30 seconds on each leg
- ❑ **Calf stretch** (→ p. 134), 2 sets of 20 seconds on each leg

GOAL 2: STRENGTHEN AND TONE YOUR ABDOMINALS

- ❑ **Leg extension** (→ p. 64), 2 sets of 10 reps

- ❑ **Bicycle** (→ p. 68), 2 sets of 15 reps
- ❑ **Crunch, feet on the floor** (→ p. 52), 2 sets of 10 reps

GOAL 3: STRENGTHEN AND SHAPE YOUR BUTTOCKS

- ❑ **Leg lift to the side** (→ p. 76), 2 sets of 10 reps on each leg
- ❑ **Leg lift on the belly** (→ p. 78), 2 sets of 15 reps on each leg
- ❑ **Bridge** (→ p. 88), 2 sets of 15 reps
- ❑ **Leg extension to the side** (→ p. 100), 2 sets of 20 reps on each leg

GOAL 4: STRENGTHEN AND SHAPE YOUR LEGS

- ❑ **Good morning with a bar** (→ p. 116), 2 sets of 10 reps
- ❑ **Standing calf raise** (→ p. 130), 3 sets of 15 reps
- ❑ **Standing knee raise** (→ p. 106), 3 sets of 15 reps on each leg
- ❑ **Wide-leg squat** (→ p. 114), 2 sets of 10 reps

PROGRAM 2 **INTERMEDIATE**

GOAL 1: SLIM YOUR WAIST AND STRETCH YOUR BODY

- ❑ **Sphinx** (→ p. 72), 3 sets of 30 to 40 seconds
- ❑ **Buttocks stretch** (→ p. 96), 2 sets of 30 seconds on each leg
- ❑ **Static stretch for the waist** (→ p. 38), 3 sets of 20 seconds
- ❑ **Standing side bend** (→ p. 40), 3 sets of 15 repetitions on each side

GOAL 2: STRENGTHEN AND TONE YOUR ABDOMINALS

- ❑ **Sit-up, feet on the floor** (→ p. 56), 3 sets of 15 reps
- ❑ **Oblique crunch, legs raised** (→ p. 62), 3 sets of 20 reps

- ❏ **Reverse crunch** (➜ p. 66), 4 sets of 10 reps
- ❏ **Crunch, feet on a bench** (➜ p. 58), 3 sets of 10 reps

GOAL 3: STRENGTHEN AND SHAPE YOUR BUTTOCKS

- ❏ **Leg lift with a bent knee** (➜ p. 82), 3 sets of 20 reps on each leg
- ❏ **Leg lift on the knees** (➜ p. 80), 3 sets of 15 reps on each leg
- ❏ **Bridge** (➜ p. 88), 2 sets of 30 reps
- ❏ **Lateral leg curl** (➜ p. 102), 3 sets of 20 reps

GOAL 4: STRENGTHEN AND SHAPE YOUR LEGS

- ❏ **Body-weight squat** (➜ p. 108), 3 sets of 20 reps
- ❏ **Wide-leg squat** (➜ p. 114), 3 sets of 20 reps
- ❏ **Forward lunge** (➜ p. 120), 3 sets of 15 reps on each leg
- ❏ **Good morning with a bar** (➜ p. 116), 3 sets of 30 reps

PROGRAM 3 **ADVANCED**

GOAL 1: SLIM YOUR WAIST AND STRETCH YOUR BODY

- ❏ **Lying torso twist** (➜ p. 44), 2 sets of 1 minute on each side
- ❏ **Standing hamstring stretch** (➜ p. 126), 3 sets of 40 seconds on each leg
- ❏ **Torso twist with a stick** (➜ p. 42), 3 sets of 30 reps
- ❏ **Swimming** (➜ p. 48), 3 sets of 30 reps

GOAL 2: STRENGTHEN AND TONE YOUR ABDOMINALS

- ❏ **Crunch, legs raised** (➜ p. 54), 4 sets of 20 reps
- ❏ **Crunch, feet on a bench** (➜ p. 58), 4 sets of 15 reps
- ❏ **Oblique crunch, legs raised** (➜ p. 62), 4 sets of 30 reps
- ❏ **Side plank** (➜ p. 46), 3 sets of 30 reps on each side

GOAL 3: STRENGTHEN AND SHAPE YOUR BUTTOCKS

- ❏ **Bridge, feet on a bench** (➜ p. 90), 4 sets of 20 reps
- ❏ **Side leg raise on the knees** (➜ p. 86), 3 sets of 30 reps on each leg
- ❏ **Bridge with one leg raised** (➜ p. 92), 3 sets of 20 reps on each leg

GOAL 4: STRENGTHEN AND SHAPE YOUR LEGS

- ❏ **Deadlift** (➜ p. 110), 4 sets of 12 reps
- ❏ **Squat with a bar** (➜ p. 112), 3 sets of 30 reps
- ❏ **Wide-leg squat** (➜ p. 114), 3 sets of 20 reps
- ❏ **Step-up on a bench** (➜ p. 118), 3 sets of 30 reps on each leg

Library of Congress Cataloging-in-Publication Data

Delavier, Frédéric.
[Belles fesses et ventre plat. English]
Delavier's sculpting anatomy for women : core, butt, and legs / Frédéric Delavier, Jean-Pierre Clémenceau.
    p. cm.
1. Abdomen--Muscles. 2. Buttocks exercises. 3. Leg exercises. 4. Exercise for women. 5. Reducing diets. I. Clémenceau, Jean-Pierre. II. Title. III. Title: Sculpting anatomy for women.
  QM151.D44713 2012
  612.9'5--dc23

                    2012015057

ISBN-10: 1-4504-3475-4 (print)
ISBN-13: 978-1-4504-3475-1 (print)

This book is a revised edition of *Belles Fesses & Ventre Plat,* published in 2011 by Éditions Vigot.

Photography: © All rights reserved unless © Thinkstock. pp. 8, 33: Hemera; p. 13: Ciaran Griffin/Stockbyte; pp. 14, 23: George Doyle/Stockbyte; pp. 15, 20: iStockphoto; p. 16: Goodshoot; p. 22: Martin Poole/Digital Vision; p. 25: Comstock Images; pp. 28, 35: Polka Dot Images/Getty Images; p. 34: Jupiterimages/Pixland. **Illustrations:** © All illustrations by Frédéric Delavier unless © Thinkstock. pp. 10, 36, 50, 74, 104: Hemera. **Graphic design:** Claire Guigal. **Photoengraving:** Claire Guigal.

Human Kinetics books are available at special discounts for bulk purchase. Special editions or book excerpts can also be created to specification. For details, contact the Special Sales Manager at Human Kinetics.

Printed in France by Pollina - L61532A   10 9 8 7 6 5 4 3 2 1

Human Kinetics
Website: www.HumanKinetics.com

United States: Human Kinetics
P.O. Box 5076
Champaign, IL 61825-5076
800-747-4457
e-mail: humank@hkusa.com

Canada: Human Kinetics
475 Devonshire Road Unit 100
Windsor, ON N8Y 2L5
800-465-7301 (in Canada only)
e-mail: info@hkcanada.com

Europe: Human Kinetics
107 Bradford Road
Stanningley
Leeds LS28 6AT, United Kingdom
+44 (0) 113 255 5665
e-mail: hk@hkeurope.com

Australia: Human Kinetics
57A Price Avenue
Lower Mitcham, South Australia 5062
08 8372 0999
e-mail: info@hkaustralia.com

New Zealand: Human Kinetics
P.O. Box 80
Torrens Park, South Australia 5062
0800 222 062
e-mail: info@hknewzealand.com

E5787